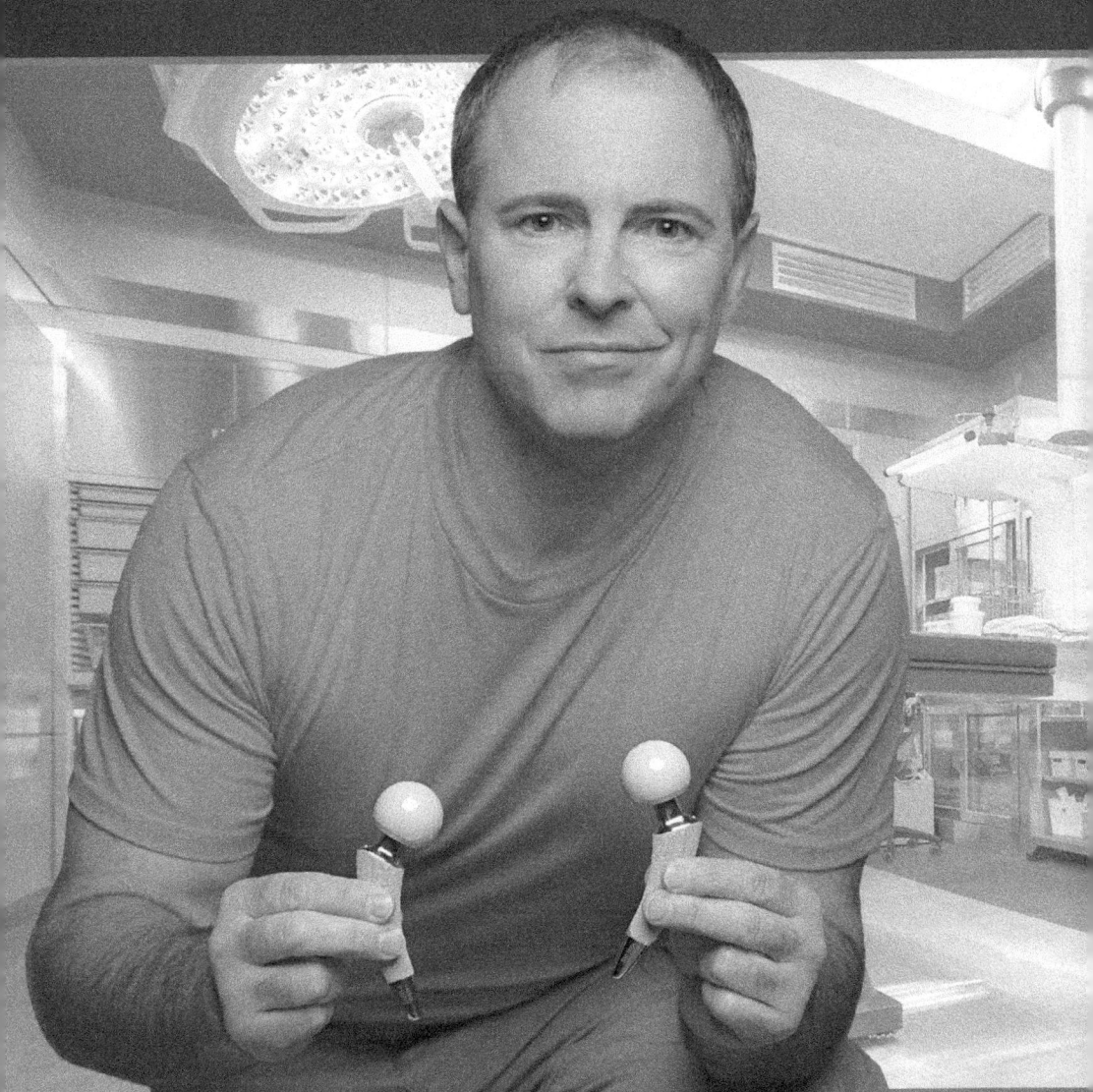

Also by Chris Bystriansky

*Renting From My 6-Year-Old*

# NEW STEEL

REPLACE DOUBT AND FEAR WITH RESOLVE AND COURAGE

FROM TWO HIP REPLACEMENTS TO TWO TRIATHLON FINISHES

## CHRIS BYSTRIANSKY

**BYSTRIANSKY GLOBAL PRESS**

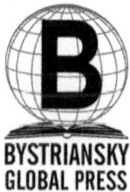

Published by Bystriansky Global Press

Cover photo by: Dean Stewart Photography

Cover and Interior Design: Dino Marino

Printed in the USA

Hardback ISBN: 978-1-956044-03-4

Paperback ISBN: 978-1-956044-04-1

eBook ISBN: 978-1-956044-05-8

October 2022

# DISCLAIMER

There are several instances of strong language in this book. The language was used to convey the strong emotions at the time described in the story. It is kept to a minimum.

This is my experience and guidance I am offering. I am not a doctor. I am not a physical therapist. I am not a triathlon coach. I do not design, manufacture, or sell hip implants. I am offering my experiences as a real-life hip implant user. As a matter of fact, I have two of them, one in each hip. I've gone through the surgeries and recoveries twice and have three perspectives on the surgeries and the outcomes. The first perspective is on having one hip replacement surgery. The second perspective relates to experiencing the surgery a second time. The third perspective is on living with two hip replacements and the accompanying challenges. In many ways, I am uniquely qualified to share information on hip replacement surgeries and recoveries because I experienced two surgeries from the inside. I know what it's like to live with severe hip pain and then to live with one implant and then two hip implants.

# SPECIAL INVITATION

I'd like to personally invite you to join our community of like-minded people from around the world who have experienced a hip replacement surgery, are facing one in the future, or have other life challenges to overcome. We get together virtually every month and share tips, offer encouragement, and celebrate the awesome things members do after surgery or after overcoming a life challenge. We welcome everyone. To learn about events and connect with me more, visit ChrisBystriansky.com.

I wish you all the success as you address and conquer your health, mobility, fitness, financial, mindset, and whatever other challenges you face. I believe in you and your ability to achieve whatever level of success you have in mind. Go big.

# DEDICATION

This book is dedicated to the many people and groups who have impacted me and continue to motivate me, including:

The entire medical community, for your mastery of the craft and all your efforts to make life better for patients around the world.

The entire triathlete community, for raising the bar on health and fitness and welcoming newcomers with open arms.

Current and future athletes who have completed, or are striving to complete, any event that pushes themselves beyond their comfort level, whether that is a local 5K run, an IRONMAN® triathlon, or any other fitness event. It doesn't matter where you start; just keep moving forward.

Hip replacement patients and their families.

Anyone who has overcome, or needs to overcome, challenges in their lives.

# CONTENTS

PREFACE ........................................................................................i

INTRODUCTION ...................................................................... vii

## PART 1

1. HISTORY ...............................................................................2
2. FORTUITOUS INJURY .........................................................7
3. WITH THAT BIKE? ............................................................. 12
4. NO COMPLAINING............................................................ 19

## PART 2

5. SURGERY #1—LEFT HIP.................................................... 30
6. REHAB............................................................................... 42
7. SURGERY #2—RIGHT HIP................................................. 50
8. THE RULE OF THIRDS........................................................ 61

## PART 3

9. HOW WOULD IT BE POSSIBLE?......................................... 70
10. TRIATHLON #1—IRONMAN TEXAS .................................. 91
11. TRIATHLON #2—IRONMAN ARIZONA................................124
12. GIVING BACK.................................................................... 156

CONCLUSION............................................................................ 164

TIME SPLITS FOR EACH IRONMAN TRIATHLON ...................... 169

TIPS FOR OVERCOMING CHALLENGES ................................................ 170

TIPS TO SUCCESS FOR HIP REPLACEMENT PATIENTS .................. 188

EXTRA ....................................................................................................... 206

QUICK FAVOR ......................................................................................... 208

GRATITUDE .............................................................................................. 209

ABOUT THE AUTHOR ............................................................................ 211

*When you have a good reason to do something,*
*all the good reasons to not do something*

*won't be able to stop you.*

–Chris Bystriansky

# PREFACE

To my reader, my friend,

Thank you very much for picking up this book. My mission in writing it was to give millions of people the hope and determination they need to live their lives to the fullest. Whether you are a hip replacement patient, contemplating the surgery for yourself or a loved one, or simply want to get better at overcoming challenges, there is a much better future waiting for you.

Based on an internet search, there are about 450,000 total hip replacements in the United States each year, and that number has been on an increasing trajectory for decades. I was one of those numbers recently . . . twice. Once in two different years.

I was lost for years before my first surgery. I didn't know what to do. I was in constant pain and didn't know where to go for help. I took pain meds almost every day. Standing up from a chair was agonizing. I had to stand up in slow motion because that was as fast as my hip would allow. Walking was a nightmare, and I would hold on to furniture or railings whenever possible to take the weight off my hip and make movement more manageable.

I couldn't believe what I heard when a doctor told me I had osteoarthritis and avascular necrosis in my left hip, both degenerative joint conditions. Osteoarthritis is a condition in which the cartilage covering the bones in joints wears away, leaving no protection, and a situation in which a bone rubs against another bone during movement. Avascular necrosis is a condition in which blood supply is cut off to the bone and the bone becomes brittle. I had both in my left hip. The cartilage was wearing away and the tip of the bone, the femoral head, was dying.

I was in my late thirties when I received the diagnosis—far too young for this to be happening to me, I thought. Hip replacement was imminent.

I fought it as best I could. I got second and third opinions. I tried physical therapy. I tried acupuncture. I tried PRP injections. I tried stem cells. All these simply delayed the inevitable, and I continued to live in pain until finally deciding hip replacement surgery was my only remaining alternative.

The pain and inability to live the way I wanted were pushing me toward the surgery. I couldn't even walk more than a few feet at a time. There was a greater need, though. Two months after the date of my first hip replacement surgery, my wife was due to give birth to our first child . . . a girl. I imagined what life would be like if I didn't have the surgery. I was barely able to walk. How would I help my wife? How could I take care of my baby girl? What kind of husband and father would I be?

As bad as my left hip was, and after exhausting all other known treatment options, I elected to have the surgery.

To say I was terrified would be an understatement. I can't stand the sight of blood. I hate getting shots, and the thought of what was going to happen was too much for me to think about. The doctor and staff reassured me I would be fine. I had no idea what that meant. All I knew was that they were going to slice my hip open, saw off a piece of my femur, and replace it with titanium, steel and ceramic components. The surgeon even invited me to watch a prerecorded surgery to calm my nerves.

Are you kidding me?

No way I was going to watch that.

I was scared as hell of not being able to walk, of not waking up after surgery, of something else going wrong, of dying. No matter how much those thoughts terrified me, the visions of not being able to play with my little girl or not being able to take her for walks were not acceptable. I decided that whatever the outcome surgery would bring, it would be better than the result of doing nothing and not being able to help my wife or take care of my baby girl. So, I moved forward with the surgery.

The weeks and months following surgery showed many small improvements. I informed my surgeon and physical therapists that I wanted excellent results and wanted to be back to 100 percent activity. I took responsibility for my rehab. I did all the exercises and all the reps that were prescribed, and then I did more. I started slowly and gently, but over time, I pushed it.

Eighteen months after surgery to replace my left hip, I had surgery to replace my right hip. It turns out that both hips were bad, one simply being worse than the other. Apparently, I was only feeling the pain in the hip that hurt more, and once the pain was gone and mobility returned, the other hip hurt all day long.

The decision to have the surgery on the second hip was much easier than the decision to have the surgery on the first hip. Making any tough decision or facing a challenge is easier the second time around. It always is. The mind can more easily comprehend what is on the other side of the decision or challenge the second time through, so the mind looks past the obstacles because it already knows the desired results are coming.

It took years to regain full strength and flexibility, but it was a strength and flexibility that I had not felt in over ten years. The pain started years before the surgeries as a dull ache and gradually built into a sharp jabbing pain with every step. You see, I was not only recovering from each of the surgeries, but I was also recovering from the many years of not being able to use my muscles and bones the right way. I wasn't moving correctly for many years because I was trying to avoid the pain when I moved. As a result, I stopped walking like humans are supposed to walk and moved in a manner that was least painful. Because of that, the muscles in my legs and hips weren't working as intended.

Following my surgeries, I no longer had to limp, so I relearned how to use my body to walk and move the correct way. It was a long recovery, but the more I recovered, the more the possibilities opened up for me.

I started walking a half mile and then a few miles at a time. I climbed the stairs instead of taking the elevator. I rode my bike. I walked on golf courses. I became as active as I wanted and noticed I was more active than people without joint replacements. I went from being the guy who had to have his hips replaced to the guy who was so active and, eventually, to the guy who did an IRONMAN triathlon.

Yes, I became so active that the thought of an IRONMAN triathlon, which once seemed so outlandish and crazy, was transformed into a legitimate goal. I used to think doing an IRONMAN triathlon, a single-day event encompassing a 2.4-mile swim, 112-mile bike ride, and 26.2-mile marathon, was for crazy people, and my automatic response for years was "no way." A few years after having my surgeries, my approach to fitness and many other areas in life changed. My automatic response of "no way" became one of exploring possibilities. I thought, *Well, I may not want to do this thing or that thing now, but if I did want to do those things, how would that be possible?* I looked for the possibilities rather than so quickly rejecting opportunities.

Not a day goes by that I do not stretch, exercise, or somehow maintain my hips. The muscles around my hips get tight, but it gives me the opportunity to stretch, take care of myself, and be thankful for the opportunities I have been given to experience the fullness of life.

The surgeries didn't kill me. On the contrary, they brought me back to life. I live now like I hadn't been capable of living for a long time.

Maybe you fit into one of these three groups: (1) hip replacement patients and their family members, (2) people interested in challenging themselves with an endurance event like an IRONMAN triathlon or who have already done so, or (3) people facing challenges in their lives who are trying to overcome them. I hope the words and concepts in this book give you the peace and confidence you need to overcome any obstacle and maximize your potential.

I wish you the best in accepting and recovering from whatever injury or challenge you may face in your life. There is always a way to make things better. You are not alone. There are many people ready to help you get to where you want to go. You are amazing and can achieve more greatness than you currently know.

I hope this book helps you achieve whatever you desire, whether it's great results after a surgery, confidence to overcome a challenge, better physical or mental strength, or just all-around happiness. I'm rooting for you.

All the best in life to you,

Chris Bystriansky

# INTRODUCTION

## 7:00 A.M.

*How the fuck did I get here?* I kept thinking to myself. I was lying on a hospital bed gurney in the pre-operating room at a major hospital system in Houston. I was being prepped for my hip replacement surgery, which was to happen in thirty minutes. The IV was already inserted into my right arm on the inside of my elbow. It was uncomfortable, but I couldn't really care about that at the moment.

I decided to have the surgery months ago, but now it's getting real. What was about to happen was inevitable. There was no turning back.

To say I was terrified would be an understatement.

I was a big, strong, athletic guy who swam, cycled, and did martial arts. Hell, I even golfed 100 holes in a day. I was in my thirties. This wasn't supposed to be happening to me.

My heart was racing.

I tried to think positive thoughts, but how could I focus on anything else than the surgery moving ever so closer?

I have to go piss, again. My wife helped me out of the bed, and I limped over to the restroom while wheeling the IV fluid stand along with me.

I could hide in the restroom. It provided a few moments of relief from the anxiety I felt out in the pre-op area.

The pre-op area had two rows of three beds facing each other, and each bed was sectioned off with large drapes hanging from the ceiling that could slide around each bed area to create a minor sense of privacy. Three of the other five beds were occupied with patients waiting for some type of joint replacement surgery—either hips or knees, I suppose. I could hear everyone talking. I hoped it would give me some relief by hearing others, but no way. It was hard to get my mind off what was coming.

I wasn't going to feel anything. The doctors assured me. I was going to be knocked out with some wonderful drugs, and I was still terrified.

I returned from the restroom, and my wife helped me back onto the gurney. It was my last walk with the defective hip. It was a disappointing walk. It would have been glorious if my last walk with both my natural hips had been to receive an award or a home run trot around the bases or to pick my golf ball out of the hole following a hole-in-one. But it was none of those. My last walk was just twenty feet from the restroom to the bed. That's it. That's life, I guess.

I tried to make small talk with my wife, who was sitting in the chair next to my bed. I asked her what she was going to do when they took me away for surgery.

Before she could answer, a nurse pulled back the curtain and introduced herself. She then started her pre-op process. She asked me a few questions—name, date of birth, and what surgery I was going to have. I felt like she was taking my dinner order rather than getting me ready for the scariest thing I had ever faced. I was anxious. No one else seemed to be bothered, though. Everyone was so matter-of-fact and business-like. They did this every day, so it wasn't a big deal to them. It was a big damn deal to me, though.

The nurse checked my IV, shaved the incision area, wrote a big X on my left hip, and walked away to see the next patient. I guess the big X is what they do to ensure they operate on the correct joint.

## T MINUS LESS THAN FIFTEEN MINUTES

Another steady stream of visitors came to see me. They included a hospital business manager (who had me sign paperwork here, here, and here), a surgery case worker to ensure I had everything I needed *(what could I possibly need at a time like this?)*, another nurse to check my IV, the surgeon to explain the surgery and timing, a supporting doctor to introduce himself, and the anesthesiologist, who was going to be my best friend for the next hour or so. I was a pretty popular guy that morning.

The surgeon explained that the surgery would last less than an hour, with about half of that spent on opening and closing me back up. It sounded like his team worked quickly. He said he had something like five or six surgeries scheduled that day, so yes, his team did move quickly.

Only an hour!

He explained the length of surgery to me months earlier during an office visit, but I still couldn't believe something so threatening to me and life-changing would be over so quickly. Heck, I've been in a dentist's chair longer than the time it would take for them to replace my hip!

The anesthesiologist was last to visit me. It was just him, me, and my wife in my little curtain-walled area. He explained that he was giving me an oral medication to calm me down, and then shortly thereafter, he would give me anesthesia through the IV to knock me out. I let him know I thought those were both great ideas. He said he was going to be with me the entire surgery and then would accompany me to the recovery room to wake me back up.

That was the best part to me, the waking-up part. It reminded me of being on an airplane. The flight may be good, but the landing is the most important part.

I tried to stay confident by telling myself that this would all be over in six months following physical therapy and that I wouldn't even notice a difference between the old hip and the new hip. I could get back on with my life. I felt I was being overly optimistic but screw it; it's all I had at the moment.

I started feeling drowsy.

## T MINUS ONE MINUTE

A nurse opened the curtain and pushed it all the way back, leaving a large opening to wheel the gurney through. She unhooked my IV from the stand and attached it to the gurney. We waited for my wife to gather our things, and then the four of us—me, my wife, the anesthesiologist, and the nurse—left the pre-op area.

The nurse pushed my gurney, and I was so tired I just laid there and watched the ceiling lights pass as I struggled to keep my eyes open. I was relieved the anesthesia was working.

My pregnant wife held my hand as she walked next to me while I was rolled down the hall on the gurney. She stayed with me as long as she could while we moved down the hallway. When we arrived at two big doors, she was to go to the waiting area.

I had no idea how this would turn out.

I hoped I was making the right decision.

I was out.

# PART 1

*The only relevant things about yesterday
are the lessons learned.*

-Chris Bystriansky

# 1

# HISTORY

When I was about six years old, I woke up early one Saturday morning and couldn't move one of my legs. I don't remember which one. It seemed as if my hip was locked, and I couldn't straighten my leg. I crawled to the living room in pain to watch the Saturday morning cartoons. I don't recall getting injured or doing anything that would have caused this. I went to bed the night before, and everything was fine. When I woke up, my hip felt locked, and I couldn't move my leg. That's all I knew.

A family friend came over to carry me to the car, and my mom drove me to the emergency room. I spent the next several days in the hospital while the doctors tried to figure out what was wrong. The doctors gave me some medications, and a physical therapist worked with me for those few days I was in the hospital. I was sent home with crutches and used them for the next week—even in school. The diagnosis was inflammation in the hip caused by a virus. I'm not sure how accurate that was. I don't know if that was part of the natural growth process, whether I sustained an injury, or whether it was the beginning of the end for my hips.

After a few weeks, my hips seemed fine, and I went about my life as if nothing had happened.

## LUNGS

I was often sick as a kid. My hip issue and the resulting emergency room visit was just one of the many occasions I was in and out of the hospital or visiting doctors. I also suffered from symptoms of asthma and routinely had severe breathing difficulties, leading to more and more doctor visits where I was given steroid shots and a host of other medications to get my breathing under control.

I also had several bouts of pneumonia. That led to more hospital stays. Today, we know that people with asthma symptoms are more likely to develop pneumonia because of compromised lung tissue. What do you suppose was used to treat the pneumonia? If you guessed more steroids, you are correct. We also know today that steroids can have a detrimental impact on joints if used at high doses or over long periods.

It turns out that my asthma was correlated with being around animals. We always had pets in our house, including dogs and cats. Whenever there were brief stints of time when we didn't have pets, my breathing improved only to get worse when animals were reintroduced. I'm not sure why nobody put two and two together to figure out what could have been the problem, but it was eventually resolved. When I was twelve or thirteen, we removed all pets from the house. My breathing improved. Even today, with strong lungs, if I find myself around some pets for an extended period, particularly cats, I can feel my breathing become slightly more labored.

## GRAINS

Another major health problem I had, which I didn't realize was a problem until later in life, was that I was intolerant to gluten, a protein in grains. My stomach discomfort had grown so severe and disruptive to my life by the time I was in my twenties that I needed answers. I had appointments with several doctors and gastroenterologists, supposed experts in this field, and they couldn't provide answers. Some "experts" said it was stress. Some even wanted to cut out portions of my intestines to investigate. By pure chance, I met an individual at a professional event, and we later connected over lunch. I noticed he was eating much differently than what I would consider normal. He explained that he previously had symptoms similar to the ones I was experiencing all the time. He referred me to a leading expert on gluten.

When I received the results of a genetic test and learned that not only was I incapable of processing gluten but that my body was treating the hundreds of different proteins, which make up the concept of gluten, as poison and creating autoimmune disorders, my eating and health history all made sense. My diet growing up consisted heavily of breakfast cereal, sandwiches, burritos, and pizza. For years I thought the stomach issues I experienced were normal. Nothing could have been further from the truth. I was eating gluten all day long, and it was causing serious underlying health issues.

Grains, in all their derivatives, are essentially poisonous to me. Imagine waking up every morning and drinking a teaspoon of bleach. The body has to address the poison being taken and is eventually going to develop problems. Would it make things any better if the bleach were baked into delicious foods like breads or cakes or put into soft drinks or sports drinks? Of course not, but since I was intolerant to gluten, it was akin to the constant negative impact my food had on my body. I only bring this up because it may be possible that my body was preoccupied with fighting this issue and unable to spend the resources to fix any damage being done to my hips.

This is the topic for a different book, but I mention it here because it contributed to my being sick as a kid. It may or may not have had something to do with my hip issues.

## WEIGHT

I was a big boy. And when I say big, I don't mean tall. I mean wide. Without being able to breathe normally and without knowing the impact of my food, I wasn't a very healthy kid. I started playing baseball when I was six years old, but other than that, I just wasn't very active. As a result, my weight continued to increase. By the time I was twelve years old, I weighed over 240 pounds. That's a lot of weight for a kid.

Throughout my childhood, I was in the vicious cycle of having difficulty breathing, eating food my body couldn't process, and carrying a lot of extra weight.

I wasn't the type of kid who appeared to have endurance events in my future. The cards were stacked against me. By all accounts, I should never have been qualified to even think about completing an IRONMAN event. I would never have been voted "Most Likely to Complete an IRONMAN triathlon" when I was growing up.

I mention the asthma symptoms, resulting steroid shots, gluten intolerance, and excessive weight as possible contributing factors for the hip issues I encountered later in life. While many people develop hip issues over time from years of wear and tear, I felt my hip issues escalating in my thirties, which is young for a person to experience the damage I did from wear and tear alone.

## THE TURNAROUND

When I was thirteen, I lost sixty pounds over the winter. I was in eighth grade, junior high. I gained speed and agility. I became a much more effective athlete. I underwent such a dramatic change that my baseball coaches, whom I'd had for the previous six summers, didn't even recognize me when summer baseball started.

By the time high school began, I was in good enough physical condition to try out for and make the hockey team despite not having the skill of most of the other players. By springtime, when baseball season started, I was in very good shape and could keep pace with all the physical conditioning, something that would have been impossible just eighteen months earlier.

Without resolving these issues—lungs, diet, and weight—I could not have contemplated an IRONMAN triathlon. Without starting to make some changes in the right direction, I would have likely had a much different experience in high school and later in life, and the skills I needed to set the foundation for an IRONMAN triathlon may not have been realized.

# 2

# FORTUITOUS INJURY

Have you ever had something terrible happen to you, but it wasn't until years later that you realized it was actually very good for you? Maybe it was ending a career path, a relationship, or an activity you could no longer do. For every door that closes, for every ending, there is a new door that opens or a new beginning. Be ready for it and embrace the change.

## HOCKEY

I was a three-sport athlete in high school. I played golf in the fall, hockey in the winter, and baseball in the spring. I also played intramural football and volleyball throughout the school year. Of all these activities, the sport I excelled at the most was baseball. I stayed active throughout the year to get ready for baseball in the spring.

I'm not reliving any so-called glory years because I believe the best years of my life are whatever I'm living rather than the years behind me, but this is important.

During my second year in high school (sophomore year), I was moved up from the junior varsity to the varsity hockey team for a few games. That was standard to get some of the younger players (like me) experience at a more competitive level. The players were bigger, and the game was faster at the varsity level.

I played defense. About midway through the game, I was out on the ice for one of my shifts. I had the puck behind my own net and moved to my left to start skating up ice. I was looking to pass the puck when a player from the other team came up from my right side and checked me. Rather than hitting me high in my upper body, which would have been standard, he hit me low, taking out my legs. My right knee buckled in. I laid on the ice in pain. The medic and coaches came to check me out. The game was over for me. My teammates helped me off the ice, and I went to the hospital emergency room. I had torn cartilage and strained ligaments on both sides of my right knee.

The following season during my junior year of high school, I played a handful of hockey games on the junior varsity team but wasn't comfortable. I mainly took the unofficial role of assistant coach on the junior varsity team. The bigger impact was that I showed up for spring baseball season on the varsity team out of shape. I didn't have a rigorous hockey season that year to keep me working out and getting stronger.

## SWIM TEAM

I worked hard during the spring baseball season and into the summer to get into shape for my last year in high school and the upcoming baseball season. I didn't want to show up out of shape again. There were off-season workouts I could do with other baseball players who weren't participating in winter sports, but the idea of doing calisthenics and running sprints all winter was not that appealing to me.

I decided to join the swim team because swimming was a winter sport and would get me out of the off-season baseball workouts. I figured since I always had fun being in a pool and was in fairly good shape, how hard could it be?

Before I go any further, I want to let you know that joining the swim team as a senior in high school, with no prior swim coaching or swim team training, is relatively unheard of. The coach, somewhat affectionately referred to as "The Admiral," even commended my courage and initiative.

Compared to other swimmers on the swim team, I was a terrible swimmer. They all had many years of competitive swim team experience, even the freshmen. I was lost most of the season. I had no idea what the drills were, what the lingo was, and certainly no idea how to actually swim. I thought swimming was having a good time in the pool and getting a little exercise by swimming back and forth across the pool between the lane lines. I didn't know anything about technique, efficiency, or proper breathing. I got a very rude awakening.

I wasn't built like a swimmer. Swimmers are usually long and lean, able to glide through the water like graceful dolphins. I was built like a football linebacker, thick and wide, and I went through the water like a school bus. I wasn't graceful, fast, efficient, or pretty to watch.

I remember morning swims. We just had to come in and swim a mile in the morning before school. I left my house each morning over the winter at about 6:00 a.m. to get to school, do the morning swim, shower, and get to school on time. Then, we'd have swim practice after school.

During practice, all I had to do was follow the swimmers in front of me back and forth across the pool. The Admiral separated the swimmers into different lanes based on our speed and ability. I was always with the freshmen. My friends on the team, who were seniors like me, were in the fast lanes on the other side of the pool. It was a very humbling experience. Even at the slowest pace, I felt there were times I almost drowned, gasping for air, during practice.

Every practice made me nervous and I was worried about keeping up. The actual swim meets were even worse. I usually finished in last place in all my races at swim meets.

## THE BENEFIT

What was happening, though, was an incredible transformation. The Admiral improved my swim stroke. He improved my endurance, lung capacity, efficiency, and overall fitness. By the time baseball season started in the spring, I was in great shape. I had some of the best endurance on the team. The calisthenics, distance running, sprints, and long practices were easy for me. The previous year, I had struggled through all those workouts. But my senior year, I breezed through all of them, even while working hard.

This also set the foundation for a lifetime of swimming. Although I didn't continue swimming daily or weekly after high school, I did swim about twenty times per year to maintain my form and a little endurance. I never went too far from being a swimmer.

That decision to join the swim team, and suffering for almost the entire season, was instrumental in my long-term fitness. I had no idea at the time that my decision to join the swim team would impact me for the rest of my life. When my hips started giving me problems later in life, I could easily return to swimming as my main form of exercise. I was never fast, but I could swim a long way and do it efficiently. I swam more consistently as my hips gave me more problems.

If I hadn't sustained that knee injury, I would have continued to play hockey and would not have joined the swim team. My enjoyment of swimming for exercise would not have been developed, and I would not have been able to maintain a level of fitness once my hips started giving me problems.

Swimming was my foundation for the IRONMAN events. Later in life, I had no concerns about the swimming. The foundation for a successful swim portion of the IRONMAN triathlons had been set thirty years before the actual events.

# 3

# WITH THAT BIKE?

When I was in law school, I worked two jobs. The first job was as a law clerk on days when I didn't have classes. The second job was as a reception desk staff person at an exclusive fitness club. I wanted the second job because I could study when not helping the members, it was within a ten-minute walk from my apartment, I worked evenings, and it allowed me to use the facilities, which included a free-weight gym, racquetball courts, and an amazing outdoor lap pool.

One early evening, I was sitting behind the reception desk trying to read, but three club members were standing in front of the reception desk having a very animated conversation, and I couldn't help but pay attention to them. They were laughing and teasing each other, giving it to each other pretty hard. They seemed excited about some event coming up. I knew all three of them from the gym but knew Embry the best and felt comfortable jumping into the conversation.

"What are you guys talking about?" I asked Embry.

"There's a bike ride coming up, and I did it last year. These two guys are doing it for the first time. I was just telling them how much they're going to be suffering, and I'm going to be laughing at them."

"It sounds like a good time," I said.

"Hey, you should do it too! There's a lot of people, and it's a lot of fun," Embry continued. "It's pretty hard, though."

That's all I needed to hear.

"I'm in," I said.

I had no details, but I was game for a fun and difficult challenge. I figured since it's just a bike ride, how hard could it be?

"It's the MS150. It's a big charity ride for the Multiple Sclerosis Society. It's 180 miles over a weekend. It's in two weeks," Embry explained.

"It's what?" I asked.

I'm not sure if I was questioning the 180 miles, that it was only two weeks away, or both. Either way, the seriousness of the event and the timing caught me off guard.

"You really thinking about doing it?" Embry asked as he and the two other guys stared at me.

"Oh, of course. Yeah, I'm in," I said.

I tried to sound confident in my response, but I was borderline terrified of what I had just agreed to do. I didn't feel like I could back out and then have to see these guys regularly at the gym. For better or worse, I was in.

After work that night, I went back to my apartment, opened the door to my closet, and stared at my mountain bike covered in clothes and other crap. I hadn't been on that thing in three years.

## INSPECTION

The next day, I bought a helmet and a pump to inflate the bike tires and went for a ride. I rode for a whopping thirty minutes and only made it eight miles. After the ten-mile ride I did years earlier, this eight-mile ride was my second-longest ever.

It was so close to the date of the event that I couldn't mail in my registration. I had to go to the local MS Society office and register. That was before the internet really took off. Not only could I not register online, but I couldn't research more about the event. Everything I learned came from word of mouth or a one-page brochure. It turns out the MS150 was a two-day bike ride, with the first day being a hundred miles and the second day being eighty miles. There were rest stops with food and drinks about every ten miles.

I saw Embry at the gym a few days later and proudly let him know I had registered and completed my first training ride. He asked what kind of bike I had. I explained that I had a big, heavy mountain bike. He offered to take a look at my bike and give some suggestions to make the upcoming ride more manageable. I accepted his offer and rode my bike to the gym the next day. He told me I had to get a bike inspection at a local bike shop before the ride. He then suggested I get smooth tires for the streets to replace the current barbed tires used for riding on grass and dirt and replace the hard plastic seat with a softer, padded one for the long ride. I thanked him for the guidance.

I found a local bike shop the following day and rode my bike there to get the work done. I opened the door and walked in, rolling my bike next to me. It was squeaking. There was one clerk behind the counter, and I was the only other person in the shop.

I explained to the clerk that I was going to ride the MS150 and was there for a bike inspection.

"You're going to ride the MS150? With that bike?" he asked.

There was a clear tone of disapproving judgment in his voice. The moment was tense, and I had a suspicion we weren't going to get along, but I wanted to play it cool and confident and not let on that I was a very inexperienced rider.

"Yeah, I'm riding the MS150, with this bike," I said.

I explained that I also wanted to get smooth tires for the road and a new seat. Without looking behind him, he pointed over his head at the different tire options available that were hanging on the wall and explained the differences. They were more expensive than I thought, but I wanted to appear like I knew what I was doing, so I selected the best, most expensive tires.

"Good choice," he said.

I felt our relationship was turning around, and I was getting some respect.

"I'll grab a set of tires and take your bike back. The saddles are along the wall over there. Just pick one out, and I'll be right back."

He took my bike and disappeared into the back room.

I learned years later that experienced riders refer to bike seats as "saddles" and not "seats."

I went over to the wall where the seats were displayed. I was shocked at the number and different styles of seats. There were over twenty different shapes and sizes. I had no idea which one to select, so I again decided on a strategy of selecting the most expensive one to show this bike shop clerk that I was a serious rider and that I meant business. I took a seat off the shelf and placed it on the front counter.

The clerk came out from the back. He looked at the seat. He looked at me. He looked back at the seat.

"Is this the seat you picked?"

"Yes," I said proudly.

"Is this seat going on your bike?"

"Yep."

"This is an awesome seat. It's expensive too. But this is a women's seat. Why don't you go back there and pick out a men's seat?"

I've never felt so embarrassed in my life. I didn't know there was a difference between men's and women's seats. My strategy totally failed. I went to select a different seat, paid for everything, and left. I went back a few days later to pick up my bike. Thankfully, that same clerk was not working, but I suspect he told everyone about me.

## THE RIDE

One of Embry's friends who was not riding had a truck and picked me up at 5:00 a.m. before picking up two others and driving us to the starting area. Traffic was backed up for miles. I never knew these types of events existed, and I was shocked to be sitting in traffic on a Saturday before the sun even came up. I was hooked before the ride even started, regardless of what the day brought. There were too many people and too much energy at the event not to have a good time.

That morning, over 6,000 participants were starting their ride from Houston to Austin, Texas. We lined up in the parking lot of a high school football stadium, and after logistics announcements, words from corporate sponsors, and the national anthem, riders were released a few hundred at a time to start their trek to Austin.

## FIRST ENDURANCE EVENT

That ride was my first endurance event. Although it wasn't timed and it wasn't a race, it covered a lot of miles and took about nine hours the first day and eight hours the second day. I finished the ride each day, but I suffered and was sore in my legs, arms, hands, and whatever the area is called that I was sitting on my new seat.

I really surprised myself by completing the ride. First, I had no idea I was capable of riding that distance. Before the event, I estimated that my maximum bike ride distance would have been about fifty miles. Second, I was totally unprepared, with almost no training or special nutrition plan for the ride.

## EYES OPEN

My eyes were opened to this subculture of cyclists. Some were serious, and some were beginners like me, but it seemed everyone was there for a good time and to raise money for the charity.

The ride was also a huge social event. Not only could you talk with people while riding, but there were rest stops about every ten miles, and people were hanging out, eating, drinking, relaxing, and waiting for friends to catch up. The overnight stop was one big tailgate party, and the festivities even picked up at the end of day two at the finish line. It was one big rolling party. I knew I was going to do it again the following year.

## TEAM CAPTAIN

The following year I did more than just register to ride. I mobilized the workforce at my corporate employer to form a team to participate in the ride. We had thirty riders, six volunteers, a budget, jerseys, and a corporate tent at the overnight location. I started the team and was team captain for only one year because I left the employer. But one of the other riders continued to lead the team as the new captain for several years before handing it off to someone else.

Eighteen years after starting the team, I received a notice from my former employer that the team had reached the $1,000,000 mark for donations to the charity, which meant that a framed team jersey and a plaque with all historical rider names would be hung on the walls of the local MS150 Office.

I attended the ceremony where the framed jersey and plaque were unveiled. It was a very rewarding experience for me, not only because the team I started ultimately raised so much money for charity but also because I was so embarrassed all those years ago in the bike shop, and yet I continued to ride and even started a corporate team the following year.

## CYCLING

I continued to ride in the event each year and, as of the writing of this book, have participated in this ride over nineteen times. I wasn't a consistent rider, training throughout the entire year, but I would spend about four months and ride over 1,000 miles before the event in April, doing training rides and upping my fitness game to get ready for the ride. Because of that annual charity ride, I started to set the foundation for a successful bike portion of the IRONMAN triathlons more than twenty years before the actual events.

# 4

# NO COMPLAINING

My father was pretty much absent in my life, but one of the things he taught me dealt with reacting to something negative. For example, when I was a teenager playing hockey, he pointed out that whenever I or someone else screwed up during a game, I would shake my head in frustration, even while the play was still ongoing. It would only take a second or two, but it was time wasted when the better reaction would have been to get back into the action and make something positive happen. He was right, but it took me a long time to accept that lesson.

There were times throughout my life when things didn't go my way. I knew what I should have done or how I should have reacted to those difficult times, but often, I fell below that standard. Instead, I focused on how I was wronged in each situation or how "unlucky" I was. I should have considered the bigger picture, how fortunate I was, and how much power I had to make my situation better.

Often, it took an external shock to get me to refocus, consider the bigger picture, and take positive action.

## CYCLING SURPRISE

I was participating in a large charity bike ride outside Austin to raise money for people living with and after cancer. The ride was very popular and had about 7,000 cyclists, including celebrities and professional riders. It was October, and a cold front came through the area, making it breezy and dropping temperatures into the fifties. I joined my friend Angela for the ride, and we decided to ride the seventy-mile route, one of the longer options available.

It was several years after my initial long endurance bike ride, and I was a fairly strong rider by then. Angela was not able to be as consistent in her training due to a hectic travel work schedule, so we both expected this route to be challenging for her.

Sure enough, halfway through the ride, Angela was hurting, and our pace was much slower than at the beginning. Our 18 miles per hour pace turned into 12 to 14 miles per hour. To make matters worse, the wind picked up, and it started to drizzle. I wasn't feeling great either, and the conditions were really messing with my head. We started complaining about the weather, how the ride wasn't fun this year, and that we should have trained more and gotten more sleep the night before. We were having ourselves a little pity party and rationalizing why our ride performance was so bad.

The complaining went on for quite some time. By mile fifty, conditions got even worse. It looked like a lot of other riders quit the ride or changed their mind about doing the longer routes because there were very few riders around us. We started the day surrounded by thousands of other cyclists, but this far into the route, we could only see a few riders in the distance ahead of and behind us.

We rode on with periods of silence and periods of complaining and cursing about the situation. Suddenly, I heard this huffing and puffing coming up from behind me. It was getting louder and louder. A man, probably in his fifties, was working really hard on his bike and passed us ever so slowly—his eyes focused on the road in front of him. He was clearly putting in more effort than we were. As he passed, I quickly glanced at him and then did a double take when he was about ten feet ahead of us.

The man only had one leg.

He was riding his bike with only one leg. Not only was he riding his bike with only one leg, but he was putting in an effort like he was trying to win something. He was giving it his all. I immediately felt ashamed of all the complaining I had been doing over the past few hours and the lousy effort I was putting forth.

I turned to Angela and said, "Wow, did you see that? That guy only had one leg. Inspiring that he's out here."

She looked back at me and said very humbly, "Yeah, amazing."

We turned our focus back to the road.

One second later, we both looked at each other. She knew what I was thinking, and I knew what she was thinking, but I said it first.

"Did that son-of-a-bitch with only one leg just pass us?"

"Yep," she said.

My admiration was replaced with anger.

"Oh, hell no!" I said to Angela. "I'm leaving you behind if I have to! I'm not letting a guy with only one leg beat me to the finish!"

She agreed, and off we went, picking up our speed. We both found more energy than we realized we had. Previously, we were too busy complaining about our situation to focus on our strengths and capabilities. It took a guy with only one leg, while we both had two capable legs, to teach us something about determination. I doubt he was complaining about the weather conditions.

Every time I get on my bike, I think about this guy who taught me valuable lessons about determination and focus without even so much as looking at me. His example spoke louder than anything he could have said.

## LONG RIDE HOME

For the first half of my career in the corporate world, I worked downtown and would often commute on a bus. In the afternoon, the bus would make several stops downtown, pick up passengers, and then go nonstop to a parking lot in a suburb west of Houston, where I lived.

One day, I was leaving work after what I considered a rough day. I actually thought it was a terrible day. I wasn't happy with my job. I wasn't happy with the company. I wasn't happy with my decision to keep doing what I was doing. I was just going through the motions day in and day out. I felt sorry for myself, and for some unknown reason, I felt helpless.

I walked without purpose, wandering to my position at the back of the line, waiting for my bus to show up. There were about twenty people in line ahead of me, and I figured I had about a 50/50 chance of getting on the next bus, depending on how many people were already on the bus when it arrived at my stop.

As I stood in line, I looked to my left at another line of passengers waiting for a different bus. I had no idea where that bus route went, possibly to a different distant suburb. The line also had about twenty people in it already.

I just waited, wondering where my bus was.

I looked back at the other line and noticed another man walk up to the back of the line. He was wearing sunglasses and was holding a stick out in front of him. He was blind.

Instantly, my outlook changed, and again, I felt embarrassed. I felt embarrassed for all the possibilities I had but was squandering my time, feeling sorry for myself as if I had no control or power to make things the way I wanted them to be.

I watched in amazement as this man followed the line, kept his spacing from others, boarded the bus, and found a seat before the bus departed.

I realized I had many capabilities and resources that I was not using appropriately. I was instantly more patient, and waiting for my bus no longer seemed like a burden. I was happy to do it.

## THE EXECUTIVE

Years after witnessing the blind bus rider, I had taken steps to improve my results. I went back to school and earned an advanced degree. I obtained a better job closer to my home on the west side of town. That made my commute short and enjoyable in my own car. I had taken control of my future and was getting good results.

While I had improved my situation from years earlier and had a much better job, the career advancement that I was led to believe was available just didn't materialize. I worked hard and contributed to the organization, but I was stagnating, which was very frustrating.

There was this one guy where I worked who always seemed to be smiling. I learned his history from our conversations and knew he had been promoted time and time again relatively quickly. Not only had he been promoted frequently, but he seemed to be offered roles in which he had little experience. He wasn't particularly smart or hard-working. Needless to say, he was an overachiever.

I found him fascinating. I liked the guy, but for the life of me, I couldn't figure out how he achieved all his success. He didn't have strong business skills, and he wasn't physically impressive. So, I sought out his advice because I wanted to know what he was doing to achieve those consistent promotions.

He explained his keys to success.

"First," he explained, "be happy and smiling all the time because people, including leaders and executives, like to be around happy people."

"Second," he continued, "never say 'no' or that something is not possible. Say 'yes' always, and then try to figure out how to make it a reality. If something is really not possible, get as close as you can to the desired outcome with a solution."

"Third," he concluded, "don't complain about problems—fix them."

The guy made it sound so simple. He certainly motivated me to try different approaches, which gave me more confidence and more patience with my employer. I wanted to try that approach. I figured if this guy could be successful, then anything was possible.

I started to take a more proactive approach to getting results. I stopped focusing on any problem I was facing and looked for ways to overcome the issue. I wanted to fix every issue I came across. That likely applied more in my personal life because I had more control in that area than in my professional life.

## THE BEGINNING OF THE END

When I started to experience problems with my hips, I figured it would be an easy fix. I thought maybe my back and hips were simply out of alignment, so I went to see a chiropractor. I explained to her that my left hip was really stiff and let her know about other issues I was experiencing. She ordered X-rays to get a better understanding of my hip structure.

I returned to the chiropractor when the X-ray results were available. She was very somber and concerned when explaining that I had osteoarthritis in my left hip. That was the first time I heard the term osteoarthritis come from a doctor.

She suggested I try physical therapy to reduce the pain, but what she told me next caught me completely by surprise. She suggested I consult with a few orthopedic surgeons because she feared my hip issue was only going to get worse. She seemed genuinely affected, having to deliver that news to me.

The news didn't sink in. I didn't believe her. I thought, *How could this be possible?* Isn't osteoarthritis reserved for people much older? I was only in my mid-thirties. It can't be. It's not such a big deal, and she probably doesn't know what she's talking about. At the time, I didn't comprehend that she was suggesting I would need a hip replacement. Maybe I just didn't want to hear her.

I didn't make any more appointments with her after receiving the news. There was nothing more she could do to help me.

I was in denial for several years while my hip pain and disruption of my lifestyle continued to worsen. I couldn't walk very far. I stopped golfing. I was taking ibuprofen daily to ease the pain. Fortunately, I was able to fall back on swimming and cycling as my primary forms of exercise, but other than that, I wasn't very active.

My wife was still connected with a classmate from business school who happened to be a pediatric orthopedic surgeon. She contacted him, and he agreed to take a look at the X-rays and provide his opinion. A few weeks later, he confirmed that I had severe osteoarthritis and would likely need a hip replacement at some point in the near future.

## TREATMENTS

I became engulfed in learning about alternative treatments and didn't spend time feeling sorry for myself or complaining. Maybe all the previous lessons I learned helped me focus on finding a solution rather than wasting my time feeling sorry for myself.

I read that acupuncture may relieve arthritis symptoms, so I scheduled appointments for that treatment. Getting stuck with so many needles felt strange, but I may have felt some relief. The pain returned, so that was not a long-term solution.

I became interested in stem cell therapy. Unfortunately, I learned that, in the United States, the ability to get treated with the highest potency stem cells was limited. Still, I wanted to try the therapy to give me some pain relief and put off a hip replacement surgery as long as possible or even indefinitely. I was still in denial of the severity of the problem.

I learned of a clinic in Colorado that did stem cell therapy and treated hip issues similar to mine. I had a virtual appointment with a doctor who confirmed the osteoarthritis and avascular necrosis diagnosis and explained the stem cell procedure to me. I flew to Denver to get the treatment. As part of the treatment, a doctor drilled into the back of my pelvis, extracted bone marrow, enriched the cells, and then injected them into my hip. I returned home and was instructed to stay off the hip for a few days and then do a series of exercises in a pool for weeks.

I really wanted this to work. I was hoping my hip would return to full health. The stem cell treatment may have provided some relief, but over time, the hip pain returned. Although this type of treatment was not a long-term solution for me in my situation, I understand there are many other injuries or conditions where better results are achieved.

I tried physical therapy. The goal was to strengthen the muscles that flow through the hip area to provide better support for the bone structure. It was not intended to be a long-term fix. It was just intended to reduce the pain and increase my mobility, which was compromised due to the severe pain.

The last treatment I tried was PRP, platelet-rich plasma. By the time I received that treatment, I had already seen an orthopedic surgeon who confirmed the diagnosis. He suggested the PRP injections to possibly buy me another three to six months on my current hip, but he also confirmed what I feared—that I would need a hip replacement soon.

My left hip was severely damaged. There was no way around it. He explained that because of the avascular necrosis, the tip of the femur, the femoral head, was not getting enough blood flow and was slowly becoming increasingly brittle. If left untreated, it might eventually crack or shatter and leave me with an uncontrolled mess in my hip.

If I scheduled the hip replacement surgery, I realized I had more control over many more elements than if I were to live with it and wait for it to fail. I could control when the surgery was done, how it was done, the surgeon I wanted to use, the materials, the process, and the recovery. Plus, I could get my affairs in order. My wife and I could also both have planned absences from work.

If, on the other hand, I didn't schedule the surgery, I ran the risk of having the hip fail at some unknown time in the future. That could lead to more hip damage and the need to have an emergency hip replacement in less than optimum conditions with an unfamiliar surgeon, uncertain techniques, materials, and unplanned disruptions to both of our work schedules.

When considering the two options, I was reluctantly on board with the surgery. It seemed like the lesser of the two evils.

The only thing left for me to do was get a second opinion, again. I scheduled an appointment with a different orthopedic surgeon, who again confirmed the diagnosis and explained his hip replacement methods to me.

I didn't realize it when I made the appointment to see the second surgeon, but I inadvertently learned that different surgeons did the surgery differently. The second surgeon described the surgery and materials that were different than the way the first surgeon described. The first surgeon would use a newer technique, including the point of entry on my hip, and would use newer materials. The second surgeon would use the traditional method, including point of entry, procedure, and materials. The alternative methods would come with different risks, limitations, recoveries, and impacts on my body.

I had to decide which approach I wanted to use. So, in deciding which surgeon to use, I was indirectly deciding many different aspects of my whole experience on the day of surgery and the long-term impact. I gained comfort in having that amount of control. I researched the different processes and materials. I liked the potential of the new process, so I decided to go with the first surgeon.

My mind was set. I took control. The decision was made, and the surgery was scheduled.

# PART 2

*Cheers to all the people who were faced with obstacles when pursuing their goals*

*and told those obstacles to go to hell.*

-Chris Bystriansky

# 5

# SURGERY #1—LEFT HIP

I slowly regained consciousness as someone called my name. It took me a few seconds to remember where I was. I was in the hospital for hip replacement surgery. I wondered if the surgery was about to start or if it was over. I then noticed pressure around my left hip. I didn't feel pain, but something was definitely different. I realized it must have been over.

Everything was calm and quiet, so I figured things went relatively well. I laid still, happy to be waking up but afraid to move. I didn't want to accidentally move the hip implant or rip open the sutures. I felt stuck to the bed. I didn't know what to do, so I just laid still.

A person was standing next to me, adjusting the IV bag, and I remembered who he was—the anesthesiologist. He really was my best friend, at least for that morning.

"Welcome back. How do you feel?" he asked.

"Okay," I said.

"You did great."

"Thanks," I said with a weak smile.

"I'll be back in a few minutes. Don't go anywhere."

*Wise guy,* I thought.

As soon as he left, a nurse came into the area to check on me and asked if I needed anything. She told me my wife would be in shortly. She checked my IV and walked away.

A few minutes later, a different nurse escorted my wife into the area. I was in a post-operating recovery room. There was space for six beds, again each separated by curtains hanging from the ceiling.

My wife sat down in a chair next to the bed.

"How are you?" she asked.

"Good."

"Can I get you anything?"

"No thanks. How long was I out?"

"About two hours."

"Did the doctor talk with you?" I asked.

"Yes. He came out when he was done with his part. He said everything went perfectly, and he would come by later today."

I just laid there, still afraid to make any adjustments. I couldn't believe it was over.

About thirty minutes later, a nurse and another staff member wheeled my bed down the hall and into an elevator. We were going to the orthopedic surgery recovery floor. The standard procedure was to spend one night in the hospital for observation and then go home the following day. I was in my room by 11:00 a.m. It had been a long day already.

## UP

Later that morning, someone came in to tell me my schedule. I didn't realize I had a schedule. My plan was to just lay in bed and watch TV. I had already been through a lot that day. The person let me know I had a full schedule the rest of the day and suggested I didn't get too comfortable.

By 1:00 p.m., I was done with lunch when I heard a knock at the door. The physical therapist walked in, introduced herself, and asked if I was ready to go for a walk.

*What? Already?*

*It was a little aggressive,* I thought. I knew they would get me active but give me a break. I just had lunch and recently gained the courage to shift my weight in the bed.

I didn't think I was ready. She was standing at the foot of my bed, so I couldn't avoid the inevitable. At some point, I was going to have to move and stand on the new hip, and if the doctors and physical therapists seemed to think it was going to happen right then and there, well then, I'll go along with it.

The physical therapist helped me slide to the edge of the bed and gently moved my legs to hang down off the bed. I felt the pressure and a slight pain in the hip. I slowly stood up by putting all my weight on my non-surgery side and then ever-so-gently put weight on the surgery side as I clutched the walker, which would be my companion for the next few weeks. I felt no pain. That's because the drugs were amazing.

The timing was perfect anyway. The last time I used my old hip and was on my feet, I walked to the restroom. Where did I go on my first walk with my new hip? You guessed it, the restroom. I slowly moved my feet one after the other while grasping the walker for support. It was a little unnerving to consider that my leg was just broken that morning, and parts of my bones were removed to make room for the new hardware.

I was extremely tentative with my steps and firmly held on to the walker. I continued walking around my room for the next ten minutes before sitting in a chair beside the bed. It was time to relax for a while.

A little before 3:00 p.m., a nurse came into my room with a wheelchair to take me to the daily group physical therapy session. With a little help, I stood up from the chair and sat in the wheelchair. The nurse wheeled me about a hundred feet down the hall and into the group therapy room.

The room had a row of reclining chairs organized in the shape of a horseshoe. The physical therapist sat in a chair in the middle of the horseshoe, and a dozen patients sat in the recliners. The session was about forty-five minutes long and included hip and knee replacement patients. I was by far the youngest patient; I'd estimate by at least twenty years.

The physical therapist and her assistants took the group through a series of gentle mobility exercises. I breezed through them. I think the exercises were designed to increase mobility and keep the blood flowing. Some of the patients were in pretty bad shape, either being severely overweight or in a lot of pain. I had it pretty good compared to them.

After the group session, I went back to my room to relax. A doctor came in to talk with me and take a look at my dressings. There was a thick bandage over the front of my left hip. The bandage, which was about the size of a half sheet of paper, looked clean and was sealed all around the edges. Underneath the bandage was the big stitching used to close the incision area.

I got out of bed a few more times the first day, each time gaining more confidence while still being cautious. The plan was to stay one night in the hospital, go to the group physical therapy the next day, and then go home in the late afternoon. My pregnant wife slept on the recliner in my hospital room that night.

## HEAVY

What did the hip implant feel like? It felt heavy. I was still very well medicated, so I didn't feel pain, but I could feel the weight. When I stood up, my balance was a little off. That could have been the medication, but I think most of the imbalance was the different weight on one side of my body. It took some getting used to.

The best way I could describe the internal feeling is like a trip to the dentist. If you've ever been to the dentist and had a cavity filled, you may have had a similar sensation. Your body knows there is something new inside you. You may have noticed a feeling of fullness or pressure in your mouth for a few days, but then as time passes, you notice the cavity filling less and less until you don't even remember it's there. It was the same way with the hip implant. My body knew there was something new inside, and it just took time to adapt enough to that feeling until it went away.

## PLASTICS AND CERAMICS

I laid in the hospital bed the evening after the surgery and wondered what type of hip I received. Not all hip replacements are equal. There are different types of hip materials and different types of procedures used to replace hips. By learning what methods and materials different surgeons use, a patient can essentially control the materials and process by deciding to use the appropriate surgeon.

In my case, I decided to use a surgeon who specialized in anterior (a frontal entry point) hip replacements. The traditional method was the posterior (a combination of side and rear entry points). Although the anterior approach was newer and fewer surgeons were practicing the method, it was supposed to result in an easier recovery with less impact on the surrounding tissue and muscles. There is simply less tissue to cut through and less muscle to displace than in the posterior method. Plus, after discussing it with a few surgeons, I concluded that I had a better chance of getting my full strength back and being able to highly torque my hips more whether I was cycling or swinging a golf club if the anterior approach were used rather than the posterior approach.

Here's where the uncertainty in my particular surgery came into play. Part of the reason I selected my surgeon was his use of the anterior approach, but another part was the use of certain materials, or potential use, of certain materials.

The hip implant has several components. The femoral stem, which included the femoral head, is used to replace the damaged portions of the femur. As part of the surgery, the femur is cut near the top, and a new femoral stem is inserted into the remaining portion of the femur. In my case, a very short, curved femoral stem comprised of a titanium or stainless-steel rod covered with a textured surface was used to adhere to the inside of the remaining femur. The short femoral stem, or mini-stem, was used to preserve as much of my original femur bone as possible, and the curved design was used to facilitate a less invasive surgery and mimic the natural hip mobility.

On top of the femoral stem was the femoral head, which resembles a ball. In my case, I knew the femoral head was made of ceramic, a very strong, dense, and smooth material. For visualization purposes of a femoral stem and femoral head, picture a round scoop of ice cream shoved on top of a fork.

The remainder of the components are those that are inserted up into the hip socket. The acetabular cup made of metal goes up into the hip socket. The cup could sometimes be screwed or cemented in place. The next piece is the liner, which goes inside the acetabular cup.

While I knew I was getting the short, curved femoral stem, the round ceramic femoral head, and the metal acetabular cup, the material used for the remaining piece was unknown to me. The remaining component was the liner that went inside the acetabular cup. It's the component that comes into contact with the round femoral head. That is the point of contact between the femoral head in the leg and the hip socket.

Traditionally, the liners were made with polyethylene, a type of plastic. More recently, ceramic liners have been used in some situations. Essentially, it is thought that ceramic liners would result in less wear and tear from the contact and friction with the femoral head, also made from ceramic, and therefore last longer than the traditional polyethylene liner.

I liked the concept of the ceramic liner and the possibility of a longer life span, but the problem was that they were not readily available and still undergoing FDA approvals. The surgeon I selected was participating in a research study in which a population of his hip replacement patients over a set period received the standard polyethylene liners while a different population of his hip replacement patients received the ceramic liners.

If I did not opt into the study, I would simply receive the polyethylene liner as part of the standard hip replacement. These liners generally do wear out over time and require another surgery to replace them or more of the hip components. I was so young, and since I needed the use of a hip for a long time, I wanted something that would last the longest.

I opted into the study, meaning that I had the potential to receive the traditional polyethylene liner, but I also had the potential to be selected to receive the ceramic liner. If I received the ceramic liner, the thought was that the liner would be more durable and offer a longer life.

It was a blind study, meaning the surgeon could not tell me if I would receive the polyethylene or ceramic liner. As a matter of fact, I wouldn't find out until years later, after the study had closed, meaning no more new patients were being admitted into the study.

## PSYCHOLOGICAL IMPACT

One of the aspects of the surgery and the aftermath that I wasn't immediately expecting was the psychological impact. It wasn't only difficult to come to terms with myself needing to have the surgery, but it was also difficult to accept.

How could I, at my relatively young age, have such a significant hip issue that I needed this surgery? I think it was my age that caused me the most concern. If I had been twenty years older, having this issue and needing the surgery would have seemed more acceptable because there would have been more natural, and explainable, wear and tear on my hips.

I felt defective. I felt as if it was somehow my fault and that I wasn't as good anymore. I have no idea where those beliefs or feelings came from, but I struggled emotionally to come to terms with them. I felt there was a negative stigma to it, which was exacerbated by my young age.

I had a hard time talking about it with the Human Resources and Health groups at my employer, who coordinated my health coverage and time away from the office. Since I was going to be away from the office for a few weeks, I informed my team, which was also difficult to do. How was I supposed to be an effective leader and a benefit to my organization? The news about my upcoming surgery spread much farther at work than I anticipated, and a few people started making comments, calling me the bionic man or that I would be able to run much faster. I just wanted to keep the news of my surgery quiet.

It wasn't until years later that my perceived negative stigma went away. That is possibly some part of the reason for wanting to push my physical therapy and return to full activity. I wanted to get rid of my limp and eliminate any sign of my hip issue. Now, when people find out I had my hips replaced, they are shocked because I have no limp and I'm not limited in my activities.

## THE FIRST TWO WEEKS

I left the hospital the day following my surgery. I was directed to go home, relax, and continue to do the light physical therapy started in the hospital. More stringent physical therapy in a clinic would start in three weeks. I was sent home with some pain medication and was to return to see the surgeon for a check-up in one week.

The doctors and nurses warned me about failing to take the pain medication on the prescribed schedule. I thought I took it right on time, but by midnight of the first night I was home, I was in severe pain. My wife phoned the doctor's office, and a new prescription was sent in immediately. She went out in the middle of the night to pick up the new pain meds. It was 3:00 a.m. before the pain subsided, and I was able to sleep.

I didn't move around too much during my first week at home. I wanted to stay relatively still to give the femur bone in my leg a good start on the healing process. I was slightly concerned about damaging the implant but much more concerned about tearing open the sutures.

We had bought a recliner two weeks earlier so I would have somewhere comfortable to sit after surgery. I did all my initial physical therapy sitting in that chair. I even slept in the chair because it was so comfortable. Plus, it was easier to get in and out of compared to a bed.

I used a walker to get around the house. I didn't go too far, just from the bedroom, where the recliner was, to the kitchen.

By day three following surgery, I couldn't stand it anymore. I had to take a shower. The guidance from the medical staff was not to worry about getting the dressing wet because it was supposed to be waterproof, but I was skeptical, so I did my best to keep the dressing dry. I didn't want the dressing to get wet and make the sutures underneath wet because I was paranoid about getting it infected. Still, I needed to take a shower. I put plastic wrap over the dressing and then waterproof tape around the sides of the plastic wrap.

The plastic wrap and waterproof tape worked like magic. I was able to get a shower every day, and the dressing remained dry each time. Taking a shower was something I took for granted before the surgery, but following surgery, I appreciated it so much. It made me feel better, and anything to brighten my spirits was beneficial.

One week following surgery, I had a doctor's appointment to inspect the surgical site and change the dressing. It was the first time I had been out of the house since returning home from the surgery, and I really enjoyed the car ride. Again, I used to take car rides for granted but not anymore. It was such a treat to get into the vehicle and go for a drive.

When the doctor removed the dressing from the front of my hip, it was the first time I saw the surgical site. The stitched-up incision was about six inches long and was raised up from where the skin was sewn together. It reminded me a little of Frankenstein's monster. It looked like a big zipper was used to close the incision. The doctor assured me the sutures looked good and that they would eventually even out and be barely noticeable.

I could still see part of the big X the nurse marked on the surgical site the morning of the surgery. The nurse putting that big X on me like she was branding cattle seemed so long ago.

I was sent home with a clean bill of health and a new dressing. My next appointment would be in one month.

By the second week following surgery, I continued to get more comfortable with my mobility. I even started sleeping on the bed rather than in the recliner. My wife helped me get in and out of bed. I was less concerned about moving the implant but still concerned about tearing the sutures. I had no idea how durable they were. I was getting more comfortable using the walker around the house, so I was up moving around more often.

Ten days after surgery, I discontinued the use of all pain medications. I continued to stay on schedule with the at-home physical therapy, doing the light physical therapy exercises twice each day while sitting in the recliner. I felt better and wanted to go faster in my recovery, but there was a balancing act I had to play between giving the remaining femur bone time to heal and integrate with the new femoral stem that was inserted and ensuring

I was getting enough exercise to reduce the risk of blood clots and minimize the build-up of scar tissue in the area. Strength and flexibility would come in the next phase of the recovery process.

While I was at home, I was just trying to be patient. I wanted to push and do more physical therapy, but I didn't want any setbacks in my recovery process. I wanted to heal as fast as possible.

As I was recovering at home, my wife was getting closer to our baby's due date. She was slowing down but was always ready to help me when I needed it. Our daughter was due in about six weeks. I wanted to be ready for her.

## NUMB

Something the doctors didn't mention to me when I was contemplating the hip replacement surgery was the fact that I would lose the sense of touch on my thigh. I had no sense of touch on the skin of my upper leg. The doctors had to move or cut through nerves when they made the incision in the front of my hip. For more than six months, I had no feeling in the skin on the front of my left thigh. The feeling has partially come back, but for the longest time, I couldn't feel anything in any pockets on that side of my body. It was strange to have keys or a phone in my pocket and not be able to feel them on my leg.

# 6

# REHAB

I took physical therapy seriously, probably much more seriously than a typical patient. I was an athlete growing up and knew, based on experience, the importance of physical therapists in fully recovering from an injury.

When I finally decided to move forward and schedule the surgery, the doctor's office gave me a long list of physical therapy location options. How did I know which location to select? Not all physical therapists are created equal or have the same specialties. The best approach, I thought, was to identify which therapy location and which specific physical therapist had the best experience in helping patients recover from anterior hip replacement surgeries, the same type I was going to have. I suspected the therapy required to recover from the anterior hip replacement was different from the therapy required to recover from the posterior hip replacement because different muscles are impacted during each procedure. The anterior hip replacement was a relatively new approach, so I suspected there were not too many therapists with deep experience in these recoveries.

I wanted to get it right, so I followed up with the surgeon for his recommendation on therapists. I told him my goal was to get back to 100 percent activity. I was just being optimistic. I didn't think that was possible, but I was going to try.

"Go next door," he instructed.

There was a physical therapy clinic in the office space adjacent to the surgeon's office. I learned the clinic director was involved with creating a therapy protocol for patients of the anterior hip replacement method, and he collaborated with the surgeon frequently. It sounded like the perfect place for me.

Rather than selecting a therapy location based on physical location, hours, availability, price, schedule, size of the clinic, or just a random choice, I made my selection based on the expertise of a specific therapist.

By week three after surgery, I was going for regular car rides just to get out of the house. Since the surgery was on my left side, I was able to use my right leg to drive. The only concern when driving was getting in and out of the car. I just took things slowly. I also transitioned from using the walker to using two crutches, which provided greater mobility.

## CLINIC PHYSICAL THERAPY

Three weeks after surgery, I was sitting in an examination room in the physical therapy clinic for an initial evaluation. The clinic was pretty cramped, with physical therapy tables and various exercise machines organized as neatly as possible around the space.

There was no physical therapy that first day. My visit only included a lot of questions and testing of leg strength in different directions. I was a little disappointed to come all the way to the clinic and not do any actual therapy. I was ready to get strong again, but I knew the therapist was developing a targeted rehab program for me. I would have to wait.

Over the next four months, I visited the clinic about twenty times. Each visit was almost an hour long and included a review of the exercises from the previous session, an introduction of new exercises, rotational stretches, and massaging of the muscles that attached in or through the hip area. My sessions started with me doing the exercises and stretches I learned in previous sessions because the physical therapist assigned to me wanted to ensure I knew how to do the exercises correctly.

It was amazing how small tweaks in a motion can impact the muscles differently. I learned how to do the exercises and stretches in the clinic and then repeated them at home daily. After each session in the clinic, I was sent home with a packet of information, including pictures and descriptions of each of the new exercises and stretches.

In week five, I transitioned from two crutches down to one. The physical therapists agreed with this after assessing my strength, balance, and walking gait. I was making great progress.

## HOME PHYSICAL THERAPY

I followed the physical therapy plan. I took a long-term approach. Rather than rushing back to a relatively active lifestyle, I was patient because I wanted to get back to 100 percent activity, even if it took me two or three times as long to get there.

For example, I wanted to get back to golfing. When I golf, it's my time to either think deeply on an issue or spend time with a playing partner in a rewarding conversation. Rather than rushing back to golf, I waited six months before swinging a club. If I was going to hit a golf ball, I wanted to hit it the way I used to hit one. After all, how was I going to hit a golf ball like I wanted to without strong hips and legs and the flexibility to create great rotational torque? I wanted to get back to golfing the way I used to do it before the pain stopped me years earlier.

I did the exercises and stretches every day at home. I even stretched extra. For the first six months, it took me well over an hour each day. I would stretch for ten minutes in the morning, do an hour of exercises in the late afternoon, and then stretch for another ten minutes before bedtime. I was getting results, so I was motivated to put in the extra time and effort.

## BACK IN THE POOL

What was the value of my previous decision to join the swim team in high school?

Swimming had been my go-to exercise for years when I wasn't able to do anything else because of the hip pain. Following my surgery, all I had to do was wait for the incision site to completely heal to avoid the risk of infection. That took six weeks. As soon as I could get back into the pool to swim, I was in. I used a common training tool, a pull buoy, placed between my legs to help keep my legs from sinking as I swam and to prevent me from kicking. Kicking would have had a negative impact on my recovery. I had great swims, and as a result, my cardiovascular health and upper body strength came back quickly.

That ludicrous decision I made twenty years before, to join my high school swim team as a senior, that one decision as a teenager at a time in my life when I probably wasn't making too many other good decisions, proved to be invaluable for the rest of my life. Out of all the millions of decisions I've made in my life, that one to join the swim team and suffer through the entire swim season has easily been one of the top five best decisions I've ever made.

## LOOP

I lived in a neighborhood with a three-quarters-of-a-mile street loop with houses on the outside of the loop and a small lake on the inside of the loop. Before the surgery, I feared I would never walk around the loop again. After my surgery, my goal was to walk around the loop. Three months removed from surgery, I finally made it around the loop. My hip was sore, but I made it. One lap around the loop became two, and then I was able to do three laps within five months. Walking around the loop was the first time I was realistically hopeful that I could eventually return to full activity.

## CONSTANT

Not a day goes by that I do not do some form of physical therapy. Since the surgery, I have been doing some form of physical therapy to make my leg and hip muscles stronger and more flexible.

I view the upper leg as five distinct areas to target: (1) the front of the leg, or the quadriceps; (2) the outside of the leg, or the IT band; (3) the back of the leg, or the hamstring; (4) the interior of the leg, or the groin, and (5) the glutes, or the butt. All these muscle areas either connect to the hip or run through the hip area, impacting the range of motion of the hip. In the early weeks and months following surgery, my goals were to increase strength and flexibility, but over time, the goals have changed to maintain strength and flexibility.

One of the main issues I constantly address is keeping the front of my leg, the quadriceps, stretched. The quadriceps are a major muscle group and the first area to tighten up on me, given all the use the muscles get in my cycling, swimming, and even walking. This muscle group flows through the front of the hip. When this muscle group gets tight, it pulls or compresses the hip joint in the front. All the components, including the acetabular cup, the liner, and the femoral head, then compress together, squeezing out any natural body fluid. The presence of natural body fluid allows the components to glide smoothly against each other. Without space for the fluid to circulate, the components rub together, creating friction and possibly excessive wear and tear. All these could have a negative impact on the lifespan and effectiveness of the hip.

To counteract this, I focus on stretches and exercises that stretch the quadriceps and those muscles that strengthen the rear of the hip, the hamstrings, and the glute muscles of the butt.

Yes, I do exercises to tighten my butt. There, I said it.

I also do rotational exercises to promote the movement of fluid around the hip joint components.

I gathered all this information on maintaining the hips based on my discussions with the surgeon and physical therapists, as well as my direct experience of putting my hips under stress and then recovery through exercise and stretching. When the fronts of my legs and hips get tight, I know how to counteract it through a series of exercises and stretches.

As an easy example, when I go for hikes, commonly four to six miles, I'll reserve a certain amount of the distance to walk backward. When walking forward, the front of my hips and quadriceps are engaged and tighten up. Walking backward, even for a short distance, works the back of the hamstrings and glutes, partially offsetting the impact on the front of my legs and hips. When the hike is over, stretching the front of the legs and hips and doing some easy rotational exercises completes the recovery and the maintenance needed to ensure there is space between the hip components, allowing the body's natural fluid to lubricate the moving hip parts.

## THE STRETCH

One of the tools I use almost daily is a foam roller. It's a hard foam piece of equipment shaped like a log and is about six inches in diameter and three feet long. I lay on top of the roller and then position, one at a time, my quadriceps on the front of my legs, IT bands on the outside of my legs, and then hamstrings in the back of my legs over the roller so I can roll back and forth. These are common stretches for runners. While laying on top and positioning the roller so that it's in contact with the targeted muscle group, I'm able to roll back and forth to soften and stretch the muscle tissue.

The problem I had was that those stretches with the foam roller only addressed three sides of my legs. There was a fourth side that I needed to stretch. So, I created a stretch where I would lay on the ground on my side and sandwich the roller between my thighs. The end of the roller was between my thighs, and the longer three-foot end stuck straight out to the side. I named that position the "Pecker Stretch" because the overall position resembled the beak of a woodpecker. That position was terrific for stretching the hard-to-reach groin and inside-thigh area.

One Saturday, I was meeting friends for an early morning round of golf. I arrived early, about 5:30 a.m., to use the fitness center to stretch. I turned the lights low because it was early and it was too bright. I grabbed the foam roller and laid down on the ground to start going through my stretching routine. I rolled the front, sides, and back of my legs.

It was time to start the Pecker Stretch.

I've gone through this routine hundreds of times at home and didn't think anything of it. As I was lying on the floor, engaged in the Pecker Stretch with the foam roller poking out from between my thighs and the lights turned down low, a gentleman walked in to use the exercise equipment. He looked at me lying on the floor with the foam roller sticking out between my legs. He paused, continued to look at me, shook his head, and then walked over to the far side of the fitness center. That's the last time I've done the Pecker Stretch in public.

# 7

# SURGERY #2—RIGHT HIP

Six months after my left hip replacement surgery, I felt pretty good, and the pain in my left hip was gone. There was still some occasional stiffness after excessive activity, but overall, my life was getting back to normal.

I started to notice some discomfort in my right hip. I went back to see the surgeon who replaced my left hip and had some X-rays taken. The X-rays came back bad. I had almost no cartilage remaining in my right hip. That meant hip replacement surgery was imminent. Maybe I was using my right side a lot while recovering from the left hip surgery, which accelerated the damage. Given the extent of the damage in my right hip, I suspected there was discomfort and pain previously, but I didn't notice it because the left hip felt worse, and I was focused on that side. Once the pain on my left side was gone, it was only then that I started to feel the pain that was growing on my right side.

*Here we go again,* I thought.

At the rate I was going, I was glad I only had two hips.

If there was an ounce of good news in all that, it's that my wife wasn't pregnant the second time around. I hated to burden her during my first surgery when she was pregnant. I wanted to take things off her mind and help her out more. Instead, she helped me more because I was recovering from the first surgery. We did have a one-year-old girl running around the house, though, so that was going to make things challenging while trying to be careful and moving around on crutches.

## STUDY

Do you remember that study I mentioned earlier that I opted into to possibly receive the ceramic cup liner rather than the traditional polyethylene liner? Well, because my second surgery was so close to my first surgery, the study was still open for candidates. That meant I could make the decision again to participate in the study or not. If I did not participate in the study, I would receive the standard polyethylene cup liner. If I did elect to participate in the study, then there was a chance I would receive either the ceramic liner or the polyethylene liner.

Given my age, I made a few bold assumptions. First, since I was so young at the time of my first surgery, my late thirties, and the ceramic cup liners were potentially expected to last longer than polyethylene, I was the perfect candidate for the ceramic liner. Second, assuming that I received the ceramic liner during the first surgery, I would also receive the ceramic liner in the second surgery. I came to this conclusion because, again, first, I was young, and the study results would be more meaningful if a candidate like me were given the ceramic liners. Second, assuming I received the ceramic liner in the first surgery, it would not have made medical sense to give me a different product the second time when the same product as the first was still available. I figured I would be given whatever I had before.

Do you think I opted into the study again for my second surgery? You bet your ass I did. The last thing I wanted was a polyethylene liner because of the wear and tear that didn't align with my goals of returning to full activity. If I didn't want to participate in the study, there was a 100 percent chance I would receive the polyethylene liner. If I did participate in the study, there was a chance (I thought a very good chance) that I would receive the ceramic liner and, therefore, the hips would be more durable and last longer.

As it turns out, my logic and presumptions were correct. I received the ceramic liners in both surgeries. I would not learn that information until over a year after my second surgery when the window of time to bring new patients into the study had closed. I was very fortunate to require my second hip replacement surgery so close to my first hip replacement surgery because I had the opportunity to get the same type of new hip. If the study had already closed for new hip replacement patients, I would not have been able to get the same hip.

## MENTAL APPROACH

The second time around, doing something initially difficult is usually easier. That was exactly the case with my second surgery. With my first surgery, I was scared and tentative, but with the second surgery, I was confident and decisive.

My attitude with the first surgery was, *I can't believe I have to do this,* but with the second, it was, *let's get this shit taken care of—I have other things I need to do with my life.* I was already looking past the surgery. I knew the surgery and recovery were just temporary points in my life, and I was already mentally putting my active lifestyle back together after the surgeries. I saw the light at the end of the tunnel.

I know there was just as much risk during the second surgery as there was during the first, but it wasn't so built up in my mind. Plus, I knew what to expect and how to recover. During the first surgery, the doctors, nurses, and staff were so calm and nonchalant about the process. Well, the second time, I knew why—because they have experienced them so often. I was only on my second surgery and was already comfortable with the whole process and ready to get on with it. They had been through hundreds, if not thousands, of these.

## DAY OF SURGERY

Some elements of the second surgery were similar to the first, but there were also some striking differences. The early morning check-in at the hospital and the visits from all the nurses and hospital staff were similar to the first time. I was also in the same pre-op area as before, with the curtains that hung from the ceiling to create a little privacy in the six individual spaces for patients. Almost everything else was different.

I just laid in bed and was perfectly calm. I talked with my wife as she sat in the chair next to me and answered all the questions from the nurses and hospital staff who visited me that morning.

Part of the morning pre-op routine was a visit from the anesthesiologist, a different one than in my first surgery, who was to explain to me the types of drugs he would be using. That is where the second surgery started to diverge from the first one.

The anesthesiologist considered himself a bit of a rock star. His confidence was a little over-the-top, which was fine with me as long as I didn't feel any pain and woke up after surgery.

"You know those drugs you received in your past surgery? Those weren't really that good, and we're going to do something different," he said.

"Okay, but I didn't have any problems with them," I said.

"I feel that those drugs leave my patients a little groggy and out of it for too long. So, rather than giving you the drugs through an IV, we're going to give you spinal anesthesia."

"What?"

"You'll get a sedative to calm you down, and then in the operating room, we'll do the spinal anesthesia, which will make sure you won't feel any pain through the surgery. After you get the spinal anesthesia, you'll get something to put you to sleep because it's probably better for everyone if you're asleep," he explained. "It will be easier to bring you out of sedation and will be less impactful to your body to do it this way. The anesthesia will only be working on the lower part of your body, which is exactly where we need it."

*Oh, what the hell? Why not?* I thought. This was going to be something different.

I received the sedative, and after about five minutes, I was completely relaxed. I was calm before, but after the sedative, I would have agreed with anything.

## T MINUS ONE MINUTE

It's go-time. A nurse opened the curtain and pushed it all the way back, leaving a large opening to wheel my gurney through. Again, I was wheeled from the pre-op room to the operating room area. My wife walked next to me until getting to the same big double doors that led to the operating rooms. Only patients, doctors, and nurses were allowed through the doors.

At that point during my first surgery, I was out, totally unconscious already. The second time around, though, I was relatively awake and aware. I was wheeled through the big double doors and into one of the operating rooms.

## OPERATING ROOM

I was still awake when they wheeled me into the operating room, which I thought was a little strange, but I was curious to see all the things going on around me. The operating room generally looked like what I imagined an operating room would look like, with big lights, equipment, and tools organized around the room. There was a lot more clutter than I expected. Imagine an operating room also being used for storage, with stacks of boxes. That is what it looked like. Maybe it was all the necessary equipment and tools for the day, but it wasn't as organized as I had envisioned an operating room. *Oh well, they know what they're doing.*

There was music playing and several people buzzing around getting things ready for my surgery, and I supposed other surgeries after mine would take place in the same room.

I got myself up onto the operating table. That was crazy. I still didn't have the spinal anesthesia to numb me from the waist down. That was coming soon. So, I was able to get myself, with the help of a nurse and anesthesiologist, onto the operating table.

*Is this normal?* I thought to myself. I felt like there should have been some more formal process but that we all were sort of *winging it.*

It seemed like I was dreaming. I sat on the side of the operating table with my legs hanging down and just looked around the room.

Although I was very relaxed from the sedative, I was alert enough to take in all the activity.

After a few minutes, the anesthesiologist told me it was time to get the spinal injection. Playtime was over. He went around behind me and gave me the injection. After helping me lay down on the table, he gave me the medication through my IV to knock me out.

## POST-OP

The next thing I knew, I was waking up in the post-operation recovery room. My wife was already sitting in the chair next to me, and there was a nurse checking on me.

"How long was I out?" I asked.

"About two hours," my wife said. "You were sleeping good."

"How did it go?"

"Fine. The doctor said everything was fine, and he would come see you later."

When I woke up, I felt pretty good. I wasn't groggy or tired. Instead, I seemed perfectly alert, as if I had taken a short nap and was ready to go about the rest of my day—what a contrast from the first surgery, where I was in a daze for hours after waking up. I guess the spinal injection was better and less invasive than the general anesthesia I was given during my first surgery. It's also possible, though, that because I was going through it for the second time, my body and mind were better prepared and more ready to get on with the recovery.

Within thirty minutes of waking up, I was already moved to my hospital room. It was 11:00 a.m. The plan was to stay in the hospital overnight and go home the next day. Lunch was ordered, and my wife and I were watching TV. After lunch, the physical therapist was to visit and get me out of bed for a walk, and later in the afternoon, I had a group physical therapy session scheduled.

As I lay in bed, I had an eerie feeling that I had just done the same thing. It felt a little like that movie *Groundhog Day*, where Phil Connors, played by Bill Murray, experiences the same day over and over. The strong memories from my first surgery were still etched in my mind, so I was just going through the motions of my memories in real time. It was déjà vu, I guess.

## FOUR MILLIMETERS

After lunch, the surgeon came into my hospital room to see me. I don't know how many hip replacement surgeries he had already done that morning, but if I had to guess, it was between four and six.

"How do you feel?" he asked.

"Good."

"Excellent. Everything went really well in the surgery. We did have a problem with the GPS that is used to match up the placement of your new hip with your other hip. We did the best we could, so it's still a pretty good match."

*What did he just say?*

Apparently, the surgeons use GPS to guide the placement of new hips to match the other hip. If the position of each hip doesn't match, the patient runs the risk of an abnormal walking gait, creating additional wear and tear on either of the hips or knees. It's a big deal.

*Well*, I thought, *it's just something I'll have to address later.* It wasn't until a few days after returning home that I noticed three scars, one on my non-surgery side hip and one on each of my legs, above each knee. The scars were from the metal pins inserted as reference points for the GPS. *Pretty high tech,* I thought. I just wished it worked that day. There were no similar scars after my first surgery, so maybe this GPS was something new.

The physical therapist entered my room in the afternoon and helped me out of bed. It wasn't a big deal because I had been through it before. I slowly slid my legs off the side of the bed and let them hang. Then I gently slid off the bed down to the ground until my feet touched the floor.

I immediately felt a difference in my legs. *This is what the surgeon was talking about,* I thought. My new right hip was not in the exact same position as my older left hip. The result was that my right leg felt longer. When I first stood up, it didn't feel like I was standing on a level floor. I felt like my left foot was in a hole.

*During my formal physical therapy, which was to start three weeks after surgery, I learned that my right leg was four millimeters longer than my left leg. That meant that my left leg was four millimeters shorter, which explained why it felt like my left foot was in a hole while standing.*

Still standing there next to my hospital bed, I couldn't get too involved with the different leg lengths. I could only process one issue at a time. I would somehow have to address the different leg lengths later. I was focused on the issue at hand, which was the new right hip.

I comfortably walked around the hospital room using a walker. Later in the afternoon, I went to the group physical therapy session. I was familiar with the exercises and breezed right through the hour-long session. I was even sitting in the same location as last time, eighteen months earlier.

## AT HOME

As I mentioned, once you have been through something difficult and need to go through something similar again, it's much easier. When I was at home following the right hip surgery, I simply repeated everything I knew to do and learned while recovering from the first hip surgery. All I had to do was follow the script. I wasn't worried. I knew what I had to do. I knew what it was supposed to feel like. I knew how long it would take. With so much uncertainty removed, things were just simpler. I wouldn't say it was easy, but the mental piece of the recovery was much more pleasant than the first time around.

My wife was just as helpful as the first time, which was miraculous because we had a sixteen-month-old girl running around. That complicated things because I had to be careful not to trip over anything she left lying around.

I was off pain medication again in less than ten days. I used a walker for a week, then two crutches for two weeks, then I was down to using one crutch for another two weeks. So, after five weeks, I was walking unassisted. I wasn't walking perfectly yet, but I was getting better each day.

I credit getting back to walking so quickly, and without a significant limp, to the at-home physical therapy I had been doing. The therapy was already part of my daily routine after my first surgery. Not only were my hips and muscles used to doing the exercises, but they also started returning to correct functioning following my first surgery and corresponding therapy. The bottom line was that after doing all the physical therapy following the first surgery and doing the exercises on both sides of my body, I had a great head start to a quick and complete recovery following my second surgery. When the time was right, about three weeks after surgery, I returned to the same clinic as before to start the structured sessions with the physical therapists.

# 8

# THE RULE OF THIRDS

There are literally (and figuratively) a lot of moving parts when dealing with a hip replacement. There are many logistical factors to consider and decisions to make, both before and after surgery. Perhaps the most important decision to make is the extent of the recovery. I decided to get the best possible outcome. I made that decision long before the surgery.

## RESPONSIBILITY

Who is responsible for the long-term results of a hip replacement surgery? Is it the surgeon? Is it the physical therapist? Is it the patient? Or could it be someone else? I will say with 100 percent confidence that I believe it's the patient's responsibility. Unless something goes terribly wrong during the surgery, I think the responsibility is squarely on the patient. That's the way I viewed the outcomes of both of my surgeries. I was 100 percent responsible for achieving the outcome I desired.

Think about it this way. The surgeon is only involved for about an hour (albeit the most important hour of the entire process). The physical therapist may be involved for ten to twenty hours over several weeks or months following surgery. The patient, however, is involved for a lifetime. I believed that whatever I did or didn't do before or after surgery would greatly impact the outcome of the hip replacement. I took control over the process and the outcome.

My accountability for the outcome started long before the surgery. After first learning that I had avascular necrosis and severe osteoarthritis, knowing that I couldn't stand on my hip without severe pain, I didn't just run out and schedule the surgery with any orthopedic surgeon. I did my research. I got five medical opinions on my hips and spoke with three orthopedic surgeons. Each surgeon described a different type of hip replacement surgery. Each described the type of surgery that they did. If I didn't speak with three different surgeons, I might not have realized there were different types of hip replacement surgeries. They were different based on the materials used, point of entry into the hip, and recovery process.

I did further research to learn more about the different techniques and materials. Based on what I wanted my recovery to be like and what I wanted to accomplish for the rest of my life, I realized there was clearly a best method and the best materials for my situation. If I had just accepted the guidance from the first surgeon I saw, I don't think it would have turned out like it did.

## RULE OF THIRDS

I mentioned the three parties that could possibly be responsible for the outcome: the surgeon, the physical therapist, and the patient. These are the three parties involved.

I know many people are involved in the long-term successful outcome of a hip replacement surgery. I understand there are many nurses, assisting doctors, physician assistants, support staff, researchers, medical implant company personnel, family, and friends who contribute to the long-term success. But for simplicity, I'm focusing on the three main parties, surgeon, physical therapist, and patient.

My basic Rule of Thirds states that the consistent positive ability to use the hip pain-free is a combination of three factors: (1) the surgeon's actions, (2) the initial physical therapy (including rest period), and (3) the ongoing maintenance of the hip and surrounding muscles through exercises and stretches.

The surgeons do great work and are highly skilled. Certainly, the surgeon has significant technical input on the outcome of the surgery, and great surgeons may do the little extra things that have an even greater impact. There is no doubt that selecting the right surgeon is critical to the long-term outcome. While the surgeon is only involved for about an hour, it is the most important single hour of the entire process because it sets the stage for the remainder of the recovery. Their involvement, however, hinges on the actions and decisions of the patient to hire them in the first place.

The physical therapists can potentially have much more time with the patient, but again, it depends on the decision of the patient to hire them in the first place. Let's say the physical therapists spend between ten to twenty total hours with a patient. During that time, the physical therapists can help the patient's muscles realign and start to work properly again, leading to long-term comfort and use of the hip without a negative impact on the nearby joints and muscles.

That brings us to the last party—the patient. The patient is the only person who can impact what happens prior to the surgery and is the party deciding to hire the surgeon and physical therapist. Those items alone give the patient incredible responsibility for the outcome of the surgery. But let's not forget the time following surgery. Really, the only time the patient has no control or responsibility is the hour or two he or she is sedated and undergoing surgery. All the patient has to do during that time is sleep. All the other times, from the months immediately before surgery and the months immediately after, as well as for the remainder of the patient's life, their actions or inactions will dictate the long-term outcome of the surgery.

All three parties have to do their part. But it's ultimately the patient who has the control and responsibility for the overall outcome. I decided which surgeon to hire. I decided which physical therapist to hire. I decided what outcome I wanted. I decided to do all the physical therapy. In making all these decisions, I took full responsibility for my outcome.

Obviously, the surgeon and patient are necessary parties, but I've learned that some patients overlook the physical therapist. When speaking with others who have had hips replaced, they say things like:

*My doctor told me I didn't need physical therapy.*
*I was told to just walk, and that was enough.*
*I'm not supposed to get physical therapy unless I have a problem later.*
*I'm not doing physical therapy.*

All these approaches just boggle my mind. My attitude was that the physical therapist was a necessary party. If I wanted to walk without a limp, regain strength and flexibility, hit a golf ball the way I wanted, live an active lifestyle, promote a long lifespan of the hip, and overall make as good of a recovery as possible, then the physical therapist was necessary.

Consider this. Before someone gets to the point of needing a hip replacement or accepting that one is necessary, there have likely been many years of a downward spiral in hip health. Unless a sudden injury required a recently healthy hip to be replaced with a prosthetic hip, the damage was progressing slowly. As the hip becomes less healthy, flexible, and fluid over time, the muscles around the hip, or flowing past the hip, start to be used improperly. Over time, likely several years, there is significant dysfunction in the muscles because a patient is either not using them or is using them improperly to move with as little pain as possible. Either way, the motions of the body and muscles have been disrupted. So, not only is it the physical therapist's role to help the patient recover from the trauma of surgery, where large muscles are moved or even cut to access the hip joint, but it's also to help the patient recover from years of misuse of the muscles around the hip.

The role of the physical therapist is significant and, unfortunately, sometimes overlooked. In my opinion, anyone avoiding physical therapy or not taking full advantage of therapy is not having the best recovery possible. They are leaving a better recovery on the table by not taking advantage of the skills of a physical therapist.

## SURGERY ORIENTATION

A few weeks before each of my surgeries, I attended a Joint Replacement Orientation class at the hospital where I was to have the surgeries. There were about fifteen people in the half-day course each time. Nurses, anesthesiologists, and hospital case workers came and explained what was going to happen on the day of surgery. It was the hospital's effort to prepare each patient. They also provided basic physical therapy movements that each patient was supposed to do leading up to their surgery. I did them each day before the surgeries because I understood the importance of the therapy. I also understood the responsibility I had to promote my ability to achieve my desired outcome.

## LOFTY GOALS

I wanted the best possible outcome. I don't know if I was trying to attain the goal of a great recovery or if I was trying to reduce the embarrassment I felt for needing to have the surgeries. Either way, I wanted a great outcome. I wasn't going to take the chance of leaving a portion of a better recovery on the table, so I did everything I could to make it happen.

When I originally had an appointment with the surgeon, he gave examples of patients being active after surgery, attempting to reassure me and ease my fears. I didn't believe him, and those stories were not as intriguing as what I had hoped to accomplish during my life. All those examples were below my previous level of activity anyway. I was very active before the pain in my hips prevented me from doing the things I wanted to do. I thought that even the best possible surgical outcome would leave me significantly below my previous peak level of activity.

I lowered my expectations for the future. I just wanted to be able to move around without pain. I wanted to play with my daughter and help my wife. Although these were incredibly valuable activities, my goals were pretty low. My goals were essentially to be able to walk pain-free and not be a burden to my family.

So, I was in this state of mind, with lowered aspirations for the future, for months leading up to the surgery and a few months following. It wasn't until I started seeing some results from the physical therapy and recovery that my physical goals became a little broader. I didn't have any aspirations to complete an IRONMAN event. That was still years away.

What I'm talking about is more like baby steps. I started to believe in the recovery. I experienced progress. I knew that as I continued to do the exercises with the physical therapists and at home, I would keep seeing better results. I did the exercises every day and by doing so, chipped away at the burden that was in front of me until the burden was overcome.

## LIMP

There was still a long way to go, but I took the next step with my goals. About four months after my first surgery, I was able to be more helpful to my wife, tend to my newborn baby girl, and even play with her on the floor. I met my initial goals. The next challenge I wanted to overcome was getting rid of my limp.

My limp was evidence that I had hip issues. Not only could other people see it, but I felt it too. I rocked from side to side when I walked. It reminded me of what I had been through, and I wanted to forget it all. I didn't just want to get rid of my limp. I wanted to destroy it.

I started to overcome my limp and walk almost normally after about six months following the first surgery, but the pain from my second hip caused me to walk with a new limp.

When going through the second surgery and initial recovery, I knew that I would be able to eventually regain mobility, help my wife, and be able to play with my daughter, just the way I did following my first surgery. The bigger issue, however, was the limp. I didn't want to be left walking that way for the rest of my life. I didn't want people asking me what happened or why I had a limp. I didn't want anyone to see my limp. I didn't want to walk that way. I wanted to walk perfectly.

Having two replaced hips was a much different ballgame. My body had two unnatural joints that were not in the exact same position as what I had grown up with. My muscles and hip joints had to learn to walk all over again.

I was still overcoming the damage from years of misuse of the muscles around the hip. The physical therapist and exercises were not only getting my hip stronger, but they were also realigning the muscles so they would work and move naturally. My goal was to walk as normally as anyone else so there would be no evidence of any hip surgery whatsoever. After a few more months of continuing the exercises, I was able to minimize and eventually eliminate the limp.

# PART 3

*Achievement doesn't come from doing things today
you were ready for yesterday.*

*Achievement comes from doing things today
you'll be ready for tomorrow.*

–Chris Bystriansky

# 9

# HOW WOULD
# IT BE POSSIBLE?

My hips and my confidence continued to improve as I consistently did the physical therapy exercises. I was getting stronger and more flexible. I returned to hitting golf balls about eight months after each surgery, but it wasn't until after my second surgery that I was able to really start swinging normally with no pain. Hitting a golf ball places a lot of torque on the hips. Once I was comfortable putting the pressure on my hips and swinging the club the way I wanted, I knew my hips were in good shape. All I had to do was stretch before and after my round of golf and I was fine. I even prefer to walk when I golf rather than using a golf cart unless I'm playing in an outing and carts are required. Walking a golf course is about a seven-mile hike. I like the exercise, and walking helps me stay loose and focused. Plus, I enjoy the peacefulness and tempo of the game better when I walk.

## MINDSET

Within a few years after my second surgery, I started to question many of my beliefs. I questioned my career, where I lived, how I exercised, and how I made money. I started spending time with highly successful people and added a few mentors to my life. I created goals for myself and started to think bigger. Previously, I often had an automatic response of "no" to doing something new. I would come up with reasons why something wouldn't work or why it wasn't possible for me. Having my hips replaced and then spending time with more successful people made me think differently. My approach to life changed. I no longer had an immediate response of "no" or "it's not possible." My new approach was to ask how something *would be* possible. Even if I didn't want to do something big immediately, I would question how it would be possible if I did want to do it.

That's a complete mindset shift. I had been closed to most new possibilities. The mindset shift allowed me to think more openly—to say "yes" to things or at least think about how to make something happen.

## FIRST (UNOFFICIAL) TRIATHLON

I continued to swim consistently for two or three days per week. Swimming was my main form of exercise. I also continued to ride in the annual MS150 bike ride, only missing the event once because of my hip surgeries. Since the ride was pretty long, covering a hundred miles on the first day and about eighty miles on the second day, I had to cycle more seriously in the months leading up to the event just to make the ride easier. Throughout the year, when I wasn't riding outside, I would occasionally ride inside on a spinner exercise bike. Without realizing it, I was laying the foundation for a future IRONMAN event.

One Saturday, I had a golf game scheduled for the late morning with some friends. I decided to get up early and go for a swim to loosen up. I swam laps for thirty minutes. I still had time left, so I jumped on an exercise bike and rode for thirty minutes. I got cleaned up and then walked seven miles while golfing.

I felt pretty good afterwards. I later realized that I had done a rudimentary triathlon comprised of a swim, a bike ride, and a walk. I don't exactly know why, but I started researching triathlons, including the IRONMAN triathlon. What exactly was the full event? What were the distances? What were the time limits? What were the rules? I mistakenly thought participants would be disqualified if they sat down during the event, stopped swimming, got off their bikes, or walked instead of running. It turns out that none of those were true. There's no requirement to run at all—in any triathlon. All that is required is to meet the time cutoffs.

I learned that the rules of an IRONMAN triathlon were pretty basic. In most events, participants had seventeen hours to complete the course. During the 2.4-mile swim, participants could wear a wetsuit in certain conditions, which helped with buoyancy, had to finish within about two hours and twenty minutes, and could even rest by holding onto one of the available boats or kayaks.

*I could do that,* I thought.

There wasn't even a requirement to swim any particular way. Freestyle was the norm, but nothing prevented a participant from doing the backstroke, breaststroke, butterfly, sidestroke, or any other style. Participants could even dog paddle if they wanted, as long as they met the time cutoff. I realized there was no *one way* to do an IRONMAN triathlon.

The bike course was 112 miles, and participants could rest whenever they wanted and even walk any portion of it as long as they had their bike with them. Participants had to finish the bike segment within ten hours and thirty minutes after starting their swim. I had already done about twenty-five rides of a hundred miles, so this wasn't much longer.

*I could do that,* I thought.

The marathon course was 26.2 miles. I had never done anything near a marathon distance, but there was no separate time cutoff for the marathon segment. That was probably the most shocking discovery. As long as the participants finished the entire course in seventeen hours, they could cover the marathon segment as slowly as they wanted. I learned later that the official Athlete Guide for the event even states, "Athletes may run, walk, or crawl the marathon course." That meant that as long as a participant completed the swim and bike segments quickly, more time could be left for the marathon segment.

It was eye-opening because I had initially dismissed the thought of completing an IRONMAN event as I was unwilling to run 26.2 miles and put that much pounding on my hips. Since running was not required, it became something of interest.

*I could probably do that,* I thought.

While each segment was manageable, the IRONMAN triathlon requires each to be done consecutively on the same day. I could wrap my head around two of the three segments, but the marathon was the biggest question mark, and combining all three was unchartered territory for me.

Ten years prior, I would have dismissed the idea and convinced myself that people who did IRONMAN triathlons were crazy and that I was not interested in it. I no longer had my automatic "no" response. Although it all sounded very difficult, my new attitude was, *How would it be possible for me to do an IRONMAN triathlon?*

I eliminated my original understanding of the event and the requirements. By removing my false limiting beliefs and comparing my experience and strengths against the requirements of an IRONMAN event, I started to believe it was possible.

As the months passed by, I thought more and more about an IRONMAN event. I was swimming, cycling, walking, and doing my physical therapy. Honestly, I was sick and tired of it all. I needed something else to keep me motivated. I needed a goal. Since I was doing these activities, I figured I might as well go a little bit further and create a lifetime memory by doing an IRONMAN triathlon.

Why not me? Because I have two replaced hips? That's just an excuse and the easy way out. That's bullshit. And if I'm making excuses for this, what else am I currently making excuses for, and what will I make excuses for the rest of my life?

I was in. I had to develop a strategy to be fast enough in the swim and on the bike to make up for a slower marathon time. My goal was simply to finish within the seventeen-hour time limit.

## REGISTRATIONS

In November 2018, I signed up for IRONMAN Arizona, which was to take place in November 2019. I had heard that it was a good event for a first-timer. I had a year to train.

To prepare for IRONMAN Arizona, I spoke with coaches and other experienced triathletes to gain some of their knowledge. They suggested I do shorter trial triathlons as part of my preparation. There are other shorter triathlons known as sprint triathlons, Olympic-length triathlons, and even IRONMAN 70.3® events, which are half the distance of IRONMAN triathlons.

I had other ideas. Registering for shorter triathlons wasn't appealing to me, and I didn't think that doing a shorter event would prepare my mind or body for an IRONMAN triathlon any more than doing the standard long swim, cycling, and walk sessions I was already doing. Plus, my second daughter was born in 2018 and I wasn't interested in being away from my family to participate in more events.

I decided I wasn't going to do any shorter triathlons.

Over the winter, I received an email about the upcoming IRONMAN Texas in April 2019. I figured what better way to prepare for my upcoming IRONMAN Arizona than to do a practice IRONMAN triathlon! Yes, I signed up for an IRONMAN triathlon as a training event for another IRONMAN triathlon. It was a local event for me, so logistically, it was simple to attend. I signed up for the upcoming IRONMAN Texas, which was only about four months away.

My goal was to finish one IRONMAN triathlon, so I planned to go as far as I could at IRONMAN Texas in the spring, learn from it, and then be fully ready for IRONMAN Arizona in the fall. If I finished IRONMAN Texas, that would have been a bonus, and maybe I wouldn't even bother going to Arizona later in the year.

## DEFERRALS

In March 2019, one month before IRONMAN Texas, I started to get nervous. I was working hard and doing my own thing as far as training but not following a set program. I bought into the crowd telling me I needed all types of training and practice. Unfortunately, I convinced myself I wasn't ready, so I deferred my triathlon entry to the following year, April 2020. Only later did I realize how ridiculous that decision was.

IRONMAN events allowed athletes a one-time deferral of their registration to the following year. That makes sense if the athlete cannot participate in the intended event. I figured I could take more time to train, so I might as well take it. Since I was allowed a deferral, what would be the harm in putting it off? After all, I wanted to be fully prepared, right?

The same thing happened later in the year for IRONMAN Arizona. I deferred my entry until the following year's triathlon, scheduled for November 2020.

## CANCELLATIONS

What was the harm in deferring my entries from 2019 to 2020? COVID happened. I trained hard in the back half of 2019 and into 2020 to get ready for IRONMAN Texas in April 2020. After spending hundreds of hours training for my original dates in 2019, I spent several hundred more hours preparing for the April 2020 event, only to have it canceled one month before the event due to COVID. My registration was moved to April 2021.

I took time off from training in March and April 2020 and engaged more with my wife and kids. It was great to spend more time with them. Pools were closed anyway, and people were avoiding getting together.

Over the summer of 2020, I picked back up with my training only to have IRONMAN Arizona canceled one month before the event date of November 2020. My registration was moved to November 2021.

I reduced my training schedule in November and December 2020 to save time while maintaining strength and endurance. I increased my training again in January 2021 to prepare for IRONMAN Texas in April 2021. Yet again, the event was canceled one month before the planned date in April 2021. My registration was moved to the rescheduled event date later in the year, in October 2021.

I again reduced my training for a few months before ramping it back up . . . again, over the summer. The way the schedule was at the time was that I had two IRONMAN events in the fall of 2021, just six weeks apart. While I was disappointed by all the cancellations, the schedule now lined up much better for me. I could ramp up my training one more time and cover both triathlons. Plus, I enjoyed training in the heat over the summer to prepare for fall events much more than I enjoyed training in the cold over the winter to prepare for spring events.

If all this starting and stopping is confusing, the tables below show the original dates, revised dates, cancellations, and eventual actual dates.

| IRONMAN TEXAS—DATES (REGISTERED JANUARY 2019) | | | |
|---|---|---|---|
| Planned Date | Result | New Date | Comments |
| 2019—April | Deferral | 2020—April | Voluntary Deferral |
| 2020—April | Canceled | 2021—April | COVID |
| 2021—April | Canceled | 2021—October | COVID |
| 2021—October | Finished | - | - |

| IRONMAN ARIZONA—DATES (REGISTERED NOVEMBER 2018) | | | |
|---|---|---|---|
| Planned Date | Result | New Date | Comments |
| 2019—November | Deferral | 2020—November | Voluntary Deferral |
| 2020—November | Canceled | 2021—November | COVID |
| 2021—November | Finished | - | - |

## TRAINING

Almost three full years had lapsed from the time of my original IRONMAN event registration in November 2018 to my first actual triathlon in October 2021. I ramped my training up and down several times over that period. I had no intention of training for an IRONMAN event for that long. I did a lot of things during the training, only some of which were conventional. I did a variety of things to prepare myself physically and mentally. I even did some things just to break up the monotony of the training.

I continued to swim on a semi-consistent basis. It was challenging in the winter because the pool I used was outdoors, and the heater was broken about 50 percent of the time each winter. I often had to find other pools to use just to get some swims in.

I considered joining a Masters swim group and went to try one out. These are semi-recreational adult swim programs led by a coach. When I showed up, the coach asked me what my fitness level was. Without listening to my response, he put me in a lane with beginner swimmers. Although I had not been in a pool in six weeks, I swam 3,000 meters in under an hour without stopping. I didn't go back after my trial, mainly because the night practices didn't fit in with my family schedule.

## BREATHING

One of the challenges I had to overcome was breathing on both sides when I swam. Even though I swam in high school and swam recreationally for twenty years, I always breathed on my left side. I figured I would need to learn to breathe on my right side as well because in an open water swim during the IRONMAN event, there would be times when I would need to be looking to my right or left and would need to breathe on a specific side to get calmer water. For example, if there were swimmers on my left side, I would want to breathe on my right side so as not to get waves in my mouth. Also, for sighting purposes, to be able to swim in a straight line in a lake, I would need to be able to breathe and see on both sides.

It took me about twenty sessions in the pool to get comfortable breathing to my right. It was like learning to swim all over again. My timing and rhythm while breathing on my right side were terrible in the beginning, but over time, I became more and more comfortable. As it turns out, breathing on my left side resulted in a longer and smoother stroke; when I breathed on my right side, I had a more powerful stroke. I developed the habit of using both sides in all my training sessions. What was once difficult became easy.

## SATURDAY MORNING RIDES

Although I cycled somewhat seriously for about four months a year to prepare for the annual MS150, I needed more consistent miles at higher speeds to prepare for an IRONMAN event. I met a group of riders from a local bike shop and joined them on their Saturday morning rides. The group was usually between eight and sixteen riders. We would meet at the bike shop, ride about forty miles out, and then ride back to the shop. All of them were good riders, and some were even former professionals. The owner of the bike shop even rode pretty often. She was good. I picked up some useful skills along the way, including speed drills for strength, bike handling, and accelerating through turns rather than slowing.

The hardest part of riding with that group was the start of our ride. We'd roll out of the bike shop parking lot, and then the front riders wouldn't waste any time with a warm-up. They would start off pretty fast, about 21–22 miles per hour. I found myself struggling because that's pretty fast to begin with. After I rode often enough and became one of the regulars, I started trying to get to the front to lead the group, at least for the first few miles. That way, I could control the start pace, which I liked to set at about 18–20 miles per hour. I consider that a much more gentlemanly start than the aggressive pace others would set. Once warmed up my way, I would maintain the more aggressive pace that others would set.

## 4X4X48

I heard about a Navy SEAL, David Goggins, and read his book *Can't Hurt Me.* David Goggins has an extensive military training career and an impressive endurance event resume. One of the concepts he discusses is that we as individuals can accomplish way more physically than we think we can. He suggests that when we think we are done and we have nothing left to give physically, we have only reached about 40 percent of our capacity.

One of the training exercises he described was something he called the 4x4x48. The concept is to cover four miles, every four hours, for forty-eight hours. If you're doing the math, that's forty-eight miles in forty-eight hours with likely very little sleep. When you're not moving to cover the four miles, you're welcome to sleep, eat, exercise, or go about your day, but the clock is ticking for two straight days, day and night.

I liked that concept. I wanted to incorporate it into my training with the goal of getting stronger mentally. The problem I had was that whenever I did an extended or difficult workout, my hips and quadriceps got really tight, compressing the front of my hips together, and I needed to stretch them. I was concerned about the length of the event and the amount of pounding my hips would take in a short amount of time without giving the hips and muscles time to stretch. I knew I couldn't run the challenge, but I could walk it. I would rather modify and push my limits than make up an excuse as to why I couldn't do it at all.

It was still a significant test with all the miles, lack of sleep, staying on schedule, and overcoming the mind games. Waking up in the middle of the night to do four miles is tough.

In March 2021, after the latest string of IRONMAN event cancellations, I did the 4x4x48. I started at 6:00 a.m. and did my subsequent four miles at 10:00 a.m., 2:00 p.m., 6:00 p.m., 10:00 p.m., 2:00 a.m., 6:00 a.m., 10:00 a.m., 2:00 p.m., 6:00 p.m., 10:00 p.m., and 2:00 a.m.

Each four-mile set took me about an hour. There were trails near my house where I mapped out a four-mile loop. I did the challenge there during the day, but at night, I stayed in my neighborhood doing multiple laps of a mile loop.

The first day was somewhat easy, despite covering twenty miles. I blocked off my calendar and knocked out each four-mile session. It got real the first night at 2:00 a.m. I had just fallen asleep about an hour earlier when my alarm sounded. I didn't want to get up, but I forced myself to ensure I started my next set at 2:00 a.m. sharp. That is where the mind games started. It would have been really easy to quit. I could have believed it was a ridiculous idea and just stopped and stayed in bed. I got up and kept going, though. I wanted to see if I could finish the challenge.

Outside at night, there were more mind games. I stayed in my neighborhood but kept hearing noises and seeing things move in the darkness. Maybe they were real, and maybe they weren't. I don't really know.

The next day was a little easier as far as the mind games, but I was exhausted. After my set at 10:00 a.m. the second day, I was thirty-two miles into the challenge. The second night was worse than the first with the mind games. My neighborhood was next to a forested area with a big feral pig population, and it was common for large groups of twenty or more pigs to come out at night and dig up everyone's lawns looking for food. The pigs can get pretty big, over a few hundred pounds, and I was constantly looking over my shoulder, trying to stay alert so as not to find myself in a bad situation.

I was delirious when I finished at about 3:00 a.m. on the final day. Forty-five hours had elapsed since I started the challenge, and I had slept only five total hours.

I knew it would be difficult, but it was much harder than I had thought. I felt the physical impact all over my body. I was tired, but it was the mental impact that changed my approach to workouts.

I've ridden many hundred-mile bike rides and had recently completed a marathon, but this was significantly more difficult. Those other events were completed in about six hours, but this took much longer.

## RECALIBRATE

The challenge helped me recalibrate what was acceptable or what was tolerable. I used to limit what I thought was insane or simply too much physically or mentally. I realized that I was capable of so much more and that I was not operating anywhere near my peak capabilities. As a result, I found myself doing things I would have dismissed years earlier.

Years ago, when I started working with a triathlon coach, the coach asked if I could make it to a swim session at 5:30 a.m. I remember laughing at the thought of getting out of bed early enough to get into a pool by 5:30. Now, that's standard behavior. It's my norm.

There was one occasion when I couldn't sleep at night. Rather than skipping my scheduled swim in the morning, I got out of bed earlier than expected and went to the pool. Despite only a few hours of sleep, I swam 4,000 meters before 6:00 a.m. That's an IRONMAN triathlon length swim. Having that specific experience would prove invaluable later.

I do other uncomfortable activities to keep myself disciplined and the bar high. For example, I do cold plunges during the winter. The pool complex I use has two pools, only one of which is heated in the winter. Before I get into the heated pool in the mornings, I jump into the cold pool. I've even been in the Pacific Ocean early in the morning in January before swimming some pool laps while on vacation.

On my most recent MS150 bike ride, I increased my mileage from the official 100 miles to 115 miles on the first day. My longest ride before that was 112 miles, and I wanted to finish the day with something bigger than my previous record.

## 29029

After training for so long for the IRONMAN events and having them canceled time and time again, I was worn out. I was mentally and physically exhausted. I needed something different to help me refocus.

I heard about another type of endurance event, which excited me because it was a new experience. It sounded unreasonable, which, believe it or not, was appealing to me. Remember my new attitude: Rather than an immediate "no," it was, "how would that be possible for me?"

The name of the event, 29029, represents the elevation of Mt. Everest, 29,029 feet, the highest point on Earth. The concept is that participants gather at the base of a ski mountain, hike up, take the gondola down, and repeat the process until they have ascended the cumulative height of Mt. Everest or until the thirty-six-hour time limit has elapsed. The event started on a Friday at 6:00 a.m. and ended on Saturday at 6:00 p.m.

What's not to like? It's thirty-six hours, at high elevation, and hiking up a total of 29,029 feet. That would have seemed completely unreasonable a few years prior, but now it seemed perfectly normal, and I wanted in. I called the contact number, spoke with their support team, and within a week, I was registered. It was June 2021, and the event was scheduled for mid-August.

The location of the event was Snowbasin Resort outside Salt Lake City, Utah. The elevation at the base of the mountain was over 6,300 feet, and each hike up ascended more than 2,300 feet and covered 2.3 miles. It would take thirteen hikes to attain the accumulated elevation of Mt. Everest. There were almost 250 other participants.

To put it into perspective, the average marathon takes about four hours. The average IRONMAN triathlon takes about twelve hours. The average ultramarathon (one hundred miles) takes about twenty-four hours. The average finishing time for 29029 (thirteen ascents) was twenty-nine hours. It was a tough event. I lived just above sea level in the Houston area and knew I would have trouble with the altitude. But I was still excited to give it everything I had.

• • •

## INJURY

In July 2021, one month before the 29029 and three months before my first IRONMAN event, I tore the meniscus in my left knee. I had been training really hard, and on a day when my legs were exceptionally sore, I guess I pivoted a little too quickly and I immediately felt the tear. It hurt pretty bad. I couldn't walk; I couldn't straighten my leg; I couldn't even stand on it. An MRI confirmed the tear, and I spent a week laid up, using crutches to get around and icing the knee every chance I could.

If I elected to have surgery to repair the tear, I was done with everything for the year. I had trained for years and would have missed the IRONMAN events and the 29029. If I did not have surgery to repair the tear, I would have to contend with two replaced hips and the meniscus tear. If my decision to defer my IRONMAN triathlon entries looked bad before, it just got worse because I had doubts about participating in anything.

When the swelling went down after a week, I assessed the situation. I could walk a little, but I couldn't extend my left leg, so my strides got shorter. I was able to ride the bike, but again, I couldn't extend my leg like I wanted for maximum power and comfort. I was able to swim, but I couldn't kick, so to keep training, I used a buoy between my legs to help them float.

How was I going to mitigate the knee issue so I could complete the upcoming events?

Previously, I was prepared to run a portion of the marathons during the IRONMAN triathlon if I had to in order to finish before the time cutoff, but that was no longer an option. Even worse, being unable to extend my left leg meant taking shorter strides, which meant more steps, more prolonged contact with the ground, more impact on my feet and legs, and a longer marathon time.

I had a decision to make. Do I withdraw from any or all the events because of the knee injury, or do I mitigate the issue as much as possible and move forward? Given that I had trained for so long due to all the cancellations, I wasn't willing to come up empty-handed. I decided to move forward with all the events.

While I could still do some preparation, my training went way down at a time when it should have been increasing. For example, my running and walking distance in June was close to a hundred miles, but my mileage in July was less than ten. More importantly, my feet were not as tough and prepared as they were months or even years earlier.

• • •

I knew I would have issues with the torn meniscus in my left knee during the long thirty-six-hour 29029 event. I mitigated the knee issue as much as possible by taking it slowly, using short strides, wearing a compression sleeve on my knee, and relying heavily on hiking poles, which were standard for participants.

As I got tired into the night, I slowed my pace going up the mountain even more, to be careful with my knee. There were several steep sections. When I started slipping and felt my knee twist, I decided to call it quits for the night. I finished the ascent I was on, which was my seventh for the day, at 1:00 a.m. and then put ice around my knee for an hour before hitting the showers. I wanted to protect the knee as much as possible so I could do more ascents in the morning and still do the upcoming IRONMAN events.

The complete lack of energy on the mountain was something I had never experienced before. I wasn't in pain. My spirits were good, but I had no energy. I also took extra time to stretch the front of my hips after each ascent. The uphill hiking made my quadriceps and hips tight, which compressed the joints. I had to make sure they were stretched and fluid as much as possible.

After a good night's sleep, I did three more ascents on Saturday before the end of the thirty-six-hour time limit. I made it up the mountain a total of ten times, ascending over 22,000 feet. That's probably more ascending than I'd done in the previous two years combined. At the time I was living in the Houston area, about 100 feet above sea level, and there was no real elevation anywhere. I've never done anything like that before in my life, so I don't consider any part of it a failure. That was a valiant effort of which I am certainly proud. It was an incredible experience and great training for my upcoming events.

The following year, in August 2022, I was back on the mountain at the event. I finished all thirteen climbs and ascended the full 29,029 feet. There is something symbolically rewarding about hiking up a mountain. The adversity, pushing through limits, and reaching new heights were applicable to everything I did all year long. The mountain intimidated me the first year and then I couldn't wait to get back on it the second year.

## BEING READY

When I was younger, I often thought I needed to be ready before starting anything. I thought preparation was the key to success. It wasn't until later in life that I learned that *doing* was the key to success. I held the concept of being "ready" to a high standard that I could only achieve after completing a defined amount of preparation. I rationalized not moving forward and *doing* by believing I needed more preparation before I would be "ready" to start *doing*.

I've wasted so much time in my life preparing. I've realized that failure is possible even with extensive preparation, and success is possible even with minimal or no preparation. Preparation does not guarantee success, and lack of preparation does not guarantee failure.

I didn't need to be ready. I just needed to make up my mind. I needed to start *doing*.

You can always prepare more. It's the same as basic math. You can always add one more to any number. You can always add one more training session, one more mile, one more mental session, one more rest day, one more this, one more that, or one more anything. You could have started training sooner or tapered sooner. There is always one more thing to think of to get closer to being more prepared and ready. But the truth is, there is no such thing as perfect preparation.

Being ready is a myth. You're never going to be 100 percent ready. It doesn't matter anyway. I'm not saying you shouldn't bother training or preparing for anything. I'm saying we can't wait until we believe we are fully ready to begin *doing*. We must start sooner.

I made the mistake twice of believing I wasn't ready when I deferred my original IRONMAN event entries. Look what it cost me. Rather than completing them in 2019, my events were canceled or rescheduled two and three times, and I suffered a torn meniscus before the events did occur. I'm lucky nothing more severe happened to me physically or in my life that would have prevented me from making it to the start lines. All my deferrals cost me were a few more years of training.

Finishing an IRONMAN triathlon is quite an accomplishment, for sure. In reality, though, the distance itself is relatively easy. What makes an IRONMAN triathlon difficult are the conditions—the conditions on the day of the event and the conditions under which an athlete has in their personal life.

An IRONMAN athlete, to me, is someone who doesn't just complete the distance during the event. It is someone who overcomes all the obstacles in even deciding to do an IRONMAN triathlon, makes it to the start line, and then finishes, no matter what.

I think a lot of people could complete the distance with good training and under perfect conditions. That's not how things work, though. We don't go through life under perfect conditions. An IRONMAN triathlon does not occur under perfect conditions. As any athlete who has participated in an IRONMAN event can tell you, wind, heat, cold, waves, altitude, rain, nutrition, hydration, injury, equipment, sleep, and many other obstacles are standing in the way of reaching the finish line.

There are also many other obstacles preventing people from even getting to the starting line. We need to remove those obstacles that show up before the start line, including fear, doubt, limiting beliefs, and the thought that we are not ready.

We don't have that much time left in life, and we don't know what will hit us in the future. We're going to face obstacles; we know that for sure. But, anything worth doing is worth starting. We don't have time to wait until we're fully ready.

# 10

# TRIATHLON #1— IRONMAN TEXAS

## OCTOBER 2021

There was speculation all summer that IRONMAN Texas would be canceled again. All previous cancellations were announced about thirty days before the scheduled event day. The thirty-day point for this latest scheduled IRONMAN Texas came and went without any such cancellation notices, so it appeared the event was going to be held as scheduled.

Many of the other athletes must have opted for other triathlons when given the opportunity because the number of athletes participating in this IRONMAN event was pretty small compared to IRONMAN triathlon standards. There were only between 600 and 700 athletes, while a typical IRONMAN triathlon has between

2,000 and 3,000. It was pretty small. Even dropping my gear and bike off in the designated area the day before the event, I noticed there were simply not that many bikes and, therefore, not that many athletes. I imagined this is what an IRONMAN event was like thirty years earlier, relatively small and intimate.

## TIME AND STRATEGY

I didn't train like I should. I trained like I could. My mileage was way down because I was trying to stay off my knee, but I was still sticking to my frequency of workouts. I was just spending more time and effort training for the swim and bike segments and not much on the marathon segment because that's what my body allowed.

My strategy became very important. I laid out a plan, and my goal was to stick to the plan all day. I put together a strategy with target split times for each of the three segments and pacing. I put my projected times on a little business card-sized paper, laminated it, and carried it with me on the bike and marathon segments. The information on the card helped me know where I was on timing compared to my plan. If I were too slow during a given segment, I would have to pick up the pace later.

The card was critical because I reviewed the information several times throughout the day, and it saved me from having to do too much math regarding my pace while out on the course, which can get somewhat difficult when tired. Without the cards, I ran the risk of miscalculating in my head and not making the cutoff time because of a math error out on the course.

| Swim - 7:30 | 1:30:00 | 45min/2000m | 9:00 |
|---|---|---|---|
| T1 | 0:20:00 | | 9:20 |
| Bike | 6:10 | 18mph | 3:30 |
| Bike breaks | 0:30:00 | 3 breaks | 4:00 |
| T2 | 0:20:00 | | 4:20 |
| Marathon | 7:01 | 16 min/mile | 11:20 |
| Marathon breaks | 0:30:00 | 3 breaks | 11:50 |
| | | Finish | 16:20 |

Picture of my plan on the laminated card I carried with
me on the IRONMAN triathlon bike and marathon courses

Timing was so critical for me that I wore two watches. One watch tracked the split times for all three segments plus the two transitions and the second watch just kept track of total time. I knew I would be close to the seventeen-hour cutoff time, and I couldn't risk a malfunction in one watch leaving me not knowing where I was with timing and pacing.

## TRANSPORTATION AND LODGING

The event was in The Woodlands, Texas, about an hour north of Houston, near my home. I stayed at a hotel near the triathlon start for convenience and to prevent any transportation or parking issues that could arise if I tried to drive in the morning of the event. I stayed at The Woodlands Waterway Marriott, about a hundred yards from the finish. It was also just a quarter mile from the transition area and a mile away from the swim start in nearby Lake Woodlands. The location was the most convenient option available.

## THE WOODLANDS, TEXAS

The environment was hot and somewhat humid, even in October. It was a local event, so I was used to the hot conditions. It was also windy. I had prepared all summer in those same conditions. I know there was some concern about the heat and wind among the athletes. The temperature during the bike and marathon portions was in the nineties. Generally, a peak daytime temperature of eighty degrees Fahrenheit is considered hot for a stand-alone marathon event. Unlike a stand-alone marathon, which starts in the morning, typically the coolest part of the day, the marathons in an IRONMAN event are typically completed during the hottest part of the day because they follow the 2.4-mile swim and 112-mile bike ride.

# T MINUS TWO DAYS

## ATHLETE CHECK-IN

Two days before the triathlon, I officially checked in onsite. Athletes are required to check in two days before the event. There is no check-in the next day. I suspect the point is to force athletes to arrive ahead of time, ensuring there is time to acclimate to the surroundings and to get all their gear prepared. I also suspect the local community puts out a lot of time and effort to host the event, so it's beneficial to the local community to have a large influx of revenue in hotels, restaurants, and shops over the week. There is an elevated level of excitement seeing so many athletes and spectators come together in the area over a few days leading up to the event.

Weeks earlier, I had to select a window of time to check in at the IRONMAN Village, a collection of official and merchandise tents near the finish line. There were tents where athletes checked in and tents for shopping or bike servicing. After I checked into the hotel, I walked a block to the IRONMAN Village area. I was shocked at how empty it was. I expected a lot of activity. I met up with some friends there and was able to check in hours before my designated time. The entire check-in process was laid back, and everyone was very friendly. I received my five gear bags, number (bib), timing ankle bracelet, swim cap, wristband, and bike and gear stickers, all with my athlete number on them, #528.

Every few hours throughout the day, there was an athlete briefing in the IRONMAN Village. An official standing onstage provided an overview of the rules and course descriptions to any athletes who had gathered in the area. There were about fifty athletes at the briefing I attended. We were all standing or sitting under the hot sun. That is a big no-no before an endurance event because simply being out in the heat could take a toll on the body. A few lucky folks were able to claim the limited shade areas that were available. It was at least ninety degrees. The forecast called for continued heat throughout the next few days.

I browsed around the tents, made some purchases, took pictures, and walked back to the hotel. It was all uneventful.

## WARM-UP BIKE RIDE

Typically, there are warm-up bike rides two days before the triathlon. These are usually groups of athletes who get together and ride about twenty miles to keep their muscles fresh, ensure their bikes are working properly after transportation, and get familiar with a portion of the bike course, if possible.

I didn't participate in the warm-up bike ride. I was already familiar with the terrain, and my bike wasn't transported to the event on a plane or truck, so I felt confident it was in good working order. The bike course was mostly on a toll road that was to be closed to vehicle traffic only on the event day, so there wasn't an opportunity to ride a bike on it. I had driven along the bike route on the toll road a few weeks earlier, taking note of the landmarks, road conditions, and the number and frequency of overpasses, which would require additional effort to ride up while on the bike.

Instead of a traditional warm-up bike ride, I slowly rode my bike around the marathon course, about a nine-mile loop. It was good to see the course before the actual full marathon to note any narrow or winding sections, uphills, or downhills. I was going to be on the marathon course late in the day when I was tired, so seeing it ahead of time gave me some comfort.

# T MINUS ONE DAY

## PRACTICE SWIM

There is a practice swim at IRONMAN triathlons the day before the actual event. It gives athletes the opportunity to acclimate to the water. These open water swims can present much different conditions than the body of water in which the athlete typically trains. Open water swims are vastly different than swimming in a pool, which provides smooth water, plenty of space, and great visibility. In an open water swim, the water temperature, visibility, sighting, and other nearby swimmers present different challenges.

There is also a fear or shock effect when first entering the open water. The body can tense up and hyperventilate due to the cold-water temperature, lack of visibility, the crowd of swimmers, or for a number of other reasons. The practice swim is meant to help reduce swimmer anxiety and the possible negative impact it could have on the day of the triathlon. It's a great way to acclimate to the water conditions to promote a smooth start.

The practice swim is just a short version of the actual swim course. While the full swim is approximately 4,000 meters, the practice swim may be between 500 and 1,000 meters.

I participated in the practice swim the morning before the triathlon. The swim start was in a park at the same start location as the next morning, so I got to experience the exact place of entry into the water. I noticed the "NO SWIMMING" signs posted along the waterfront but figured the event organizers got clearance and ensured some level of safety. There were several hundred people milling around the park. Some were athletes, some spectators, and others were volunteers. Since I arrived toward the end of the two-hour window for the practice swim, many athletes were already done. I put on my swimskin, a thin swimsuit that extends from the elbows to just above the knees. These kinds of suits have been used in the Olympics in the past. They don't provide any buoyancy like a wetsuit would, but they do provide more efficiency when gliding through the water than my hairy skin would. When the water is too warm for a wetsuit, many athletes opt to wear a swimskin.

Although it was just the practice swim and times were not being tracked, athletes were required to wear the ankle timing bracelet during the practice swim that they received at check-in. That promoted safety and accounted for every athlete who entered the water. Volunteers and event officials must have told me at least a dozen times at check-in and the athlete briefing to bring my timing bracelet to the practice swim. Otherwise, I wouldn't be allowed in the water. There were still some athletes trying to start their practice swims without their timing bracelets. They were turned away because they failed to bring the bracelets and, unfortunately, they didn't get a practice swim. It was unfortunate because the beginning of the swim is generally the most nervous point of the triathlon. Getting to practice that part of the event was beneficial not only to me but to many other athletes.

There was no line to start the practice swim, so once I had my swimskin on, I put the timing bracelet around my ankle, grabbed my goggles and swim cap, and headed for the water. I put one foot into the water and then the other, walking a few feet until the water was waist-deep before lunging forward and starting my swim.

I expected the water to be cold, but to my surprise, it was warmer than expected. That was only my second open-water training swim, so although I was a strong swimmer, I was still a little nervous about the whole experience. When I say strong swimmer, I don't mean fast, but I would routinely swim 10,000 meters per week in a pool.

The water was murky, and I couldn't see my hand right in front of my face in the water. I briefly felt a mild panic of hyperventilating start, but after a few deep breaths and about ten strokes, I was calm and relaxed throughout the practice swim. I tried my best to swim straight in the most efficient line possible, sighting off the shoreline and buoys, but I did stray a little offline. I'm not sure who bumped into who, but I connected a few times with other swimmers. I just figured it was great practice for the actual swim the next morning.

It was a good relaxing swim, about 800 meters. I got used to the water and the conditions, so the mission was accomplished. It was late morning, but it was pretty warm already, getting out of the water. I felt like I was on vacation, just spending time at the lake. It was a great morning.

## GEAR BAGS

Each athlete received five gear bags at check-in to use throughout the IRONMAN triathlon. Each bag had a different purpose, and athletes could access each bag only at certain points during the triathlon. Later that same day, after the practice swim, I had all five official gear bags laid out on the hotel bed, getting them ready and packed. I double- and triple-checked that I had everything I thought I needed in the bags.

I was paranoid about leaving something essential out of the bag or putting it into the wrong bag and not being able to access what I needed when I needed it. If I left something out of the correct bag, I wouldn't have access to the item during the triathlon.

The T1 Bag, or Transition 1 Bag, contained everything the athlete packed to transition from the swim to the bike segment, so it could include items like a helmet, bike shoes, sunglasses, shorts, special nutrition for the athlete, and whatever else the athlete wanted to pack and that fit into the bag.

The T2 Bag, or Transition 2 Bag, contained everything the athlete packed to transition from the bike to the marathon segments. It could include things like running shoes, a hat, shorts, special nutrition for the athlete, and whatever else the athlete wanted to pack.

The Bike Special Needs Bag contained anything the athlete would need during the bike portion of the event. It could include things like specific foods or drinks, extra inner tubes in case of a flat tire, and extra $CO_2$ canisters to inflate a tire. The Bike Special

Needs Bag could only be accessed once, and since the bike route was two loops, the athlete could access the bag at about mile marker thirty or mile marker seventy. Anything left in the bag after the bike segment would be thrown away or donated.

The Run Special Needs Bag contained anything the athlete would need during the marathon portion. It included things like specific foods or drinks, extra socks, and anything else the athlete needed to help them get to the finish line. Anything left in the bag would be thrown away or donated.

The Morning Bag was used to put personal items into before the athlete started the swim. Athletes typically arrive at the swim start in their swimsuit, shoes, and shirt and then put on their wetsuit or swimskin before entering the water. Things like cell phones, car or hotel room keys, glasses, or other personal items went into the Morning Bag, and the athlete would pick up the Morning Bag near the finish line after the event.

I went through the bags meticulously to ensure I had anything I could possibly need in the correct bag. It took hours, but I wanted to make sure I had everything. I overpacked.

## TRANSITION AREA

After spending hours getting my bags and bike ready, I carried my T1 and T2 bags and walked my bike to the Transition area about a quarter mile away from my hotel. The Transition area is the main area where athletes keep their bikes and gear for the day. Athletes passed through the area twice, the first time when transitioning from the swim segment to the bike segment and the second time when transitioning from the bike segment to the marathon segment. It could be a pretty hectic place on the day of the triathlon.

IRONMAN event rules required the athlete's bike and T1 and T2 bags to be dropped off in the Transition area the day before the event. That helped reduce the chaos on the event morning and forced the athlete to prepare in advance rather than scrambling to get things together the morning of the event.

Usually, given the large number of athletes at an IRONMAN triathlon, the bikes were kept on racks in a fenced-in area within the Transition area. The T1 and T2 bags, along with changing tents, were typically located in a separate space within the Transition area. Since this event was so small, the T1 and T2 bags were kept by each athlete's bike in the same area within the Transition space, and athletes were allowed to change gear at their bikes. I thought it was very convenient because I could access anything in my T1 or T2 bags during either of my transitions, but I understood how this would not have been possible with a larger number of athletes simply due to congestion. It was not the norm for a typical IRONMAN event.

## SLEEP

I stayed in the hotel for a total of three nights, two nights before the event and the night of the event. Even though it was a relatively local triathlon for me, I stayed in a hotel close to the event to make things logistically easier and to get acclimated to the surroundings. I slept great each night. I've heard of athletes getting very little sleep the night before the event and still performing well, but I wanted to give myself every possible advantage and one of those advantages, or perceived advantages, was to get a good night's sleep. My approach worked. I slept about seven hours each night in the hotel, which is slightly more than I get at home on a regular basis.

# T MINUS ZERO DAYS - IT'S TRIATHLON DAY!

## MORNING

After hundreds of hours and thousands of miles of training, I only had 140.6 miles left, the total distance of an IRONMAN triathlon. When I woke up, a feeling of peace came over me. There was no more endless waiting, no more days of preparation, and no doubt in my mind that I was finishing the triathlon. It was that simple. In my mind, the triathlon was over before it even started. I was going to enjoy the day and I was finishing within the time limit no matter what.

I came a long way from that day years before, lying on that hospital bed, scared and wondering what the future would hold. I succeeded at walking pain-free years earlier, and I was only hours away from starting an IRONMAN triathlon.

I was up at 4:00 a.m. and started breakfast in my room by 4:15. The swim start was pushed back to about 7:10, so I had plenty of time. I prefer to eat about three hours before an endurance event and then just have a small snack about an hour before the start.

I gathered the final items for my Bike Special Needs Bag and Run Special Needs Bag and double-checked that I had my goggles, swim cap, swimskin, ankle timing bracelet, and water bottle in my Morning Bag.

I felt like I was a little later than I had planned, leaving the hotel at 5:45 a.m., but there was a flow of athletes walking out with me. I guess my timing was fine. I walked the quarter mile to the Transition area to pump up my bike tires and add last-minute items to my T1 and T2 bags. The Transition area was very subdued. I expected a crowd, but there weren't too many athletes or volunteers around, and the music playing was somewhat somber. I was expecting more action and activity and certainly more upbeat music. Maybe it was the calm before the storm, as the cliché goes.

It was still dark outside but already warm and humid. I knew it was going to be a hot day, but I loved the feeling of it all. Walking in the dark so early in the morning to the Transition area and then to the swim start felt comfortable. Although there were other athletes making the same walk and I wasn't alone, it reminded me of the 4x4x48 I did earlier in the year. Those overnight sets prepared me for this very moment.

I didn't mind the three-quarter-mile walk. It was a good warm-up, and since there was only a single path, athletes walked over, bunched together, exchanging great words of encouragement. The good news was that we didn't have to walk back. We were going to be swimming back. The triathlon start was at one point in the lake and the exit was at another point, by the Transition area.

I was still carrying my Bike Special Needs Bag, Run Special Needs Bag, and Morning Bag. These bags were to be dropped off at the swim start, and then they would be transported to the designated points on the course for me to pick up later in the day.

As we got closer to the start and emerged from the wooded pathway to cross a bridge over the lake, I started to see the bright lights of the swim start in the distance. There were thousands of people among the athletes, volunteers, and spectators. Between all the people, lights, and loud music, it was finally the excitement I was anticipating.

## THIRTY MINUTES TO GO

I dropped off my Bike Special Needs Bag and Run Special Needs Bag but held onto my Morning Bag, which I would drop off a few minutes later after placing any last-minute items into it.

I ran into some friends who were also getting ready and met their families. After milling around the crowd for a while, I did some stretching off to the side and collected my thoughts, focusing on getting a good calm start to the day.

## TWENTY MINUTES TO GO

I was nervous but calm at the same time. I knew it was going to be a long day. There were only twenty minutes left in the more than three years of preparation. It was almost all over. The finish line for me was just twenty minutes away when I would cross the start line and take my first steps into the water.

I began changing my clothes. I had my swim shorts on under gym shorts. The gym shorts came off and I put on my swimskin, which took about ten minutes to get on properly. I took one last drink of water. My shirt, gym shorts, shoes, phone, glasses, hotel room key and water bottle went into the Morning Bag, and I dropped it off at the designated area with the volunteers. The bag would be waiting for me at the finish line later that night.

## TEN MINUTES TO GO

I self-seeded in the group of athletes under the sign that read 1:20–1:30. It meant that group of athletes was expecting to finish the swim between one hour and twenty minutes and one hour and thirty minutes. From what I could tell by all the signs displaying different swim paces, my selected pace was about in the middle. The faster paces were toward the front of the mob of athletes, and the slower paces were toward the back. The concept was to allow faster swimmers to swim at their pace and not make them swim over or around slower swimmers in front of them. Although it was a small IRONMAN triathlon by the number of athletes, it was still very crowded in the area, with athletes almost shoulder to shoulder.

## FIVE MINUTES TO GO

There were some announcements I couldn't hear. The national anthem was played as the sun rose in the clear sky. The crowd was completely silent. It was a pretty cool moment. The start was close to the bridge that I had just walked over. It was lined with spectators because it was a perfect vantage point to watch the start. I stood in the crowd of athletes, waiting. The bridge was to my left. Athletes were to enter the water and make a right turn to swim the long side of the lake.

I put my swim cap on and waited.

A few minutes later, the cannon rang out, and the first group of swimmers, the professionals, ran down the ramp and into the water. Rather than a mass swim start for the rest of the field as was customary at IRONMAN events in the past, the new protocol, due to the virus or other safety issues, was to start a small group of swimmers and then wait a few seconds before starting the next group. At that IRONMAN triathlon, groups of five swimmers were released about every five seconds. Because of my placement in the line, it would still be a few minutes before my turn to get into the water.

As I moved closer to the water, I was funneled into one of the five starting chutes separated with metal dividers. I noticed athletes in wetsuits standing along the side and not moving forward. Since this event was not "wetsuit legal" or "wetsuit optional," meaning the water was not deemed cold enough to allow athletes to wear wetsuits, these athletes still chose to wear wetsuits but would have to start last after all the other athletes who adhered to the no-wetsuit protocol. Those athletes would also not be eligible for awards if their performance would otherwise warrant it.

With less than a minute to go, I put on my goggles and inched closer to the water. A loud beep signaled every five seconds for the next wave of athletes to enter the water. I watched the athlete in front of me disappear into the water, and a volunteer held out his hand for me to wait.

The beep sounded again. It was my turn.

## SWIM

The water was warm enough. I was glad I did the practice swim the day before. There was an immediate right turn after starting the swim, so I had positioned myself on the left side of the entry chute to make a wide right turn once I got in the water to avoid being swam over or bumped at the beginning of the swim.

I felt the mild panic again soon after starting the swim but took a few deep breaths, and within about ten strokes, my breathing normalized and I was calm. I settled into a good rhythm and was intentionally swimming slower than normal because I considered it a warm-up. There was a long way to go in the swim and a long day ahead of me, so swimming fast at the start wasn't going to be beneficial. I wasn't trying to break any records. All I needed to do was swim according to plan, finish it safely, and go on to the next segment.

I did my best to sight off the shoreline and houses along the lakefront, but I ended up off-course several times. There were volunteers in kayaks and boats along the swim route to guide swimmers and keep them from getting too far off. I never needed that kind of directional help, but I wasn't really taking the most direct path either. Swimmers were allowed to stop and rest by holding onto one of the boats or kayaks as long as they didn't push off when they restarted to swim. I didn't need to take any breaks in the water.

After the immediate right turn when entering the water, the swim went along the shoreline for about 1,500 meters, took two left turns, and came back about 1,500 meters on the other side of the lake. Swimmers then took a right turn into a narrow channel and headed to the finish.

I bumped several swimmers along the way, but nothing was too impactful. We just kept going. Things got interesting in the channel because it was much narrower than the lake. There were concrete walls along the sides of the channel, and there was a slight bend to the right in the channel. I must have zoned out because I was breathing and sighting to my right, and at one point, I bumped into the wall on the left side of the channel. I wasn't paying attention to the left side and thought I had plenty of room. I didn't fully appreciate the curve of the channel. I didn't notice anything until the end of the night, but my left hand that hit the wall was cut, and the glass on my watch was cracked. My watch worked the rest of the day, so maybe that's why I didn't notice the damage. Either way, I had another watch on my right wrist to fall back on if the one on my left wrist ended up broken.

I was alternating between feeling good and relaxed on the swim and wondering when the hell I was going to be done with the swim and get out of the water. One hour and thirty minutes after getting into the water, I finished the swim and walked up the stairs, making my way to the Transition area.

## TRANSITION ONE

The Transition area was very close to the swim exit. It was only about a hundred meters from the swim exit to my bike, which was in the middle of the Transition area. Since my T1 and T2 bags were both at my bike, I had everything I needed in one location. The Transition area was fenced off, and only athletes and volunteers were allowed inside, but there were spectators along the fence, cheering for athletes.

Typically, athletes try to be in and out of Transition as quickly as possible. Many athletes grab their bikes, helmet, and shoes and leave Transition quickly, within a few minutes. They don't change clothes. They don't take any nutrition. They don't talk to anyone. They grab their bikes from the bike rack in Transition and run with them until they reach the designated area to mount their bikes and start riding.

That wasn't me. I took my time. I planned on a sixteen-hour day, so a few extra minutes in the Transition area were no big deal. Plus, it was a gorgeous day outside, so what was the rush?

I changed out of my swimskin and swim shorts into bike shorts by wrapping a big towel around my waist for privacy. There was a changing tent available, but I didn't see the need to waste time going all the way over there. Many athletes wear triathlon shorts, which can be used during the swim, bike, and run portions, or a triathlon suit, a short and shirt onesie that they wear all day. I wanted clean, dry, comfortable shorts, so I opted for the extra few minutes to change into cycling shorts and a cycling jersey. I also brushed my teeth (come on, who really wants that lake water in their mouth all day?), ate, drank, and chatted with spectators. I then walked my bike to the start of the bike course, where I was allowed to mount the bike. Fast transitions are under five minutes, but all told, I spent twenty minutes from the time I left the water to the time I started riding on the bike course. That was a long time, but I felt great.

## BIKE

The bike course was about twenty miles on main roads around The Woodlands before getting on the main portion of the bike route, which was on a major tollway running north and south from The Woodlands at the north end toward downtown Houston at the south end.

## FOOD ON THE ROAD

My cycling jersey had three pockets on the back, which I stuffed with powdered drink mixes and nutrition I knew I could eat. Since it was going to be hot outside all day, I erred on the side of caution and brought more than I would normally carry on a ride. My pockets were so full of nutrition that, at about mile ten on the ride, I reached back to grab a snack, and as I pulled it out, everything else in that same pocket came with it and scattered all over the road. I lost one-third of the nutrition and drinks I had packed but kept going because it would have been too dangerous to stop and interfere with the riders behind me while trying to retrieve everything. Plus, I packed extra nutrition in my Bike Special Needs Bag, which I could access later during the ride. I just kept riding, feeling disappointed for only a moment.

Twenty miles into the bike ride, I entered the toll road. The southbound lanes of the toll road were closed to vehicle traffic. A cement barrier, about four feet tall, separated the northbound lanes from the southbound lanes. There were portions where railroad tracks separated the northbound and southbound lanes.

I was warned that the 112-mile bike segment was so boring that seeing a freight train while out on the ride would be the highlight of the bike segment.

Once on the toll road, the route called for athletes to ride twenty miles south, then make a U-turn and ride twenty miles back, and repeat this loop before riding the remaining twelve miles back to The Woodlands on local streets. Athletes would ride their southbound and northbound routes all on the southbound lanes of the toll road, which was plenty wide for riders going in both directions.

There was no scenery on the toll road. It really was boring. The vehicular traffic on the northbound lanes of the toll road was somewhat deafening most of the route. Although on the other side of the four-foot-tall concrete barrier, the vehicles were less than twenty feet away and screamed by at eighty miles an hour, many honking their horns.

The wind was blowing from the south at about 15 miles per hour, so heading into the wind made for a difficult ride, but the wind was helpful on the return. I rode 10–12 miles per hour going into the wind and then 24–26 miles per hour with the wind. There were also a number of overpasses along the toll road, which offered short but tough climbs, especially when riding into the wind.

Wind is tough. Even though part of the ride was against the wind and part of it was with the wind, it never seems to offset completely. I've never been able to recapture all the losses of riding into the wind by riding with the wind. For example, if I normally ride 20 miles per hour but go into a headwind and slow down to 12 miles per hour, I'm not able to fully compensate by coming back with the wind along the same route at 28 miles per hour.

It was a tough ride with the strong headwind for twenty miles at a time and the short but numerous climbs up the overpasses. My legs were fairly big and strong, so they weren't in too much trouble.

Although my legs were fine, my feet were giving me concern. My feet and toes were cramping quite a bit. I was getting additional salt and potassium throughout the ride, but my feet and toes were cramping to the point of pain, and I had to get off the bike to stretch them. I had planned to make three stops at the Aid Stations but had to make two more unplanned stops to stretch my toes.

I suspected my cycling form was not optimum because the cramping in my toes and feet was accompanied by a burning sensation. I felt like I was pressing down on the pedals, putting too much pressure on the front underside of my feet, the area known as the ball of the foot. The area had been sore after cycling for a while, and I suspected some soft tissue damage might be to blame. It showed up in a big way but getting off my bike for a few minutes provided enough relief for it not to be a huge concern.

I wasn't in danger of missing any cutoff time, so it didn't bother me to stop for a few extra minutes. Little did I know that the issue would continue to get worse. I figured it was a temporary pain I could easily mitigate with a few extra breaks, so I wasn't concerned.

When I was nearing the end of the second and final loop on the toll road portion, I was riding with the wind at my back and moving pretty good. I noticed there were still riders going in the other direction, starting their second loop. They had twenty more miles going into the wind, twenty miles coming back with the wind, and then twelve more miles through the backroads to the bike finish. They looked like they were struggling, and I had some doubts if they would make the bike segment time cutoff.

I did see a freight train and waved to the conductor. It was the highlight of my ride on the toll road. Whoever told me that was right.

I exited the toll road and had twelve miles left to go to the Transition area. I felt strong over those last twelve miles and even passed some riders who appeared to be coasting into the finish. I wasn't pushing to try to shave time off or put in a personal best time. My quick pace toward the end was simply what was comfortable at the time.

I crossed the bike finish line in six hours and forty minutes, dismounted my bike, and walked it back to the rack in the Transition area. At some IRONMAN events, there are volunteers at the bike finish line, known as "Bike Catchers," who take the bikes back to the rack while the athletes go in a different direction to retrieve their T2 bags and prepare for the marathon. However, at that IRONMAN event, there were no such Bike Catchers. Given that my T2 Bag was located where I was taking my bike, I didn't really miss the perk of having a volunteer take my bike.

## TRANSITION TWO

Like the first transition earlier in the day, I took my time during the second one. There were very few athletes around because they were either still out on the bike course or already out on the marathon course. It didn't matter to me. I knew I was following my triathlon plan pretty well, and I had the time needed to have a nice enjoyable transition. Again, I changed my clothes. I wrapped a beach towel around me to change out of my bike shorts and into some dry, comfortable shorts for the marathon. I talked with a few other athletes in the Transition area. I got some nutrition, brushed my teeth, relaxed a little, and enjoyed the moment.

I was inside the fenced area by the bike and gear bags in Transition and had conversations with spectators standing along the fence. It was incredible being on my side of the fence. Rather than being a spectator, I was a participant inside the action. There's no better place to be.

Although it was a hot and sunny day, I still felt pretty good. But the sun was intense, and there was no shade nearby, so I was more motivated to get moving to get out of the sun rather than save time. Just over twenty-two minutes after dismounting my bike, I started the marathon course.

## MARATHON

The marathon course was filled with lots of spectators, different scenery, and many well-stocked Aid Stations. The course was flat, with only a bridge over a portion of the lake we swam in earlier that provided any noticeable elevation change.

The course was a nine-mile route that required three loops. Approximately one-third of the loop was pretty solitary, on trails or roads through a canopy of trees. Another one-third of the loop was through neighborhoods with multimillion-dollar homes lining the streets. The final one-third of the loop was high energy and was lined with bars, restaurants, and spectators who were there all day, having a good time.

Aid Stations were about a mile apart and staffed with very energetic and encouraging volunteers. Water, electrolyte drinks, and snacks were available.

I started my marathon in the late afternoon. It was hot, but I reached some shady areas early in the nine-mile loop. I had to walk due to the tear in the meniscus of my left knee. I didn't feel the tear all day and wanted to keep it that way. I knew that if I didn't injure it further during the marathon from a misstep or a fall, I would finish the IRONMAN triathlon within the time limit. So, I focused on taking short strides to protect my knee.

I didn't notice my hips at all. Taking the marathon slowly took a lot of pressure off my hips. I needed to ensure the joints stayed lubricated because the constant motion could easily build up friction and heat. I kept drinking liquids all day, which was beneficial because it was hot and I was sweating.

I didn't put my body under too much undue pressure. I was well hydrated, and all I had to do was keep moving forward at a steady pace. I just needed to follow my plan. I consulted my laminated triathlon strategy card and knew I was tracking the times closely, which gave me some comfort.

After putting the pressure on the balls of my feet during the bike portion, my feet were sore, and I felt them with every step. The skin and tissue on the balls of my feet were soft and not in good shape for a marathon, whether walking or running it.

When training for a marathon, it's common to put on lots of training miles. In doing so, the skin, tissue, and muscles in the feet are built up over time and can withstand the impact of the long endurance event that is the IRONMAN triathlon. That's how my feet were for the past few years as I built up my training, only to have the events canceled several times just a month before the scheduled dates. Because of the tear in the meniscus of my left knee just three months before this triathlon, I wasn't able to ramp up the training or even maintain the training I was doing to keep my feet in shape. My training miles went down significantly between the time of the injury in July and the October IRONMAN triathlon event. I was doing my best to heal the knee by staying off it, and getting my feet ready for the IRONMAN triathlon wasn't a primary consideration.

Walking a marathon sounds easier than running a marathon. It is certainly easier cardiovascular-wise because the heart doesn't have to work as hard during a walk. But walking that distance is no easy task. Strides when walking are much shorter than strides while running, and therefore walking requires the feet to impact the ground many more times. Plus, walking simply takes longer and requires more time on the feet in the heat.

My first nine-mile loop around the course was uneventful. Spectators were doing their best to encourage me to run rather than walk, but I tried to explain as best I could that it wasn't going to happen today.

The spectators were phenomenal. They cheered for everybody. The best way I can describe it is to imagine a massive tailgate party spread out along much of the nine-mile loop. I passed the time talking with other athletes and engaging with the spectators and volunteers along the way.

By the second loop, my feet were burning. I knew there was a problem. I figured the problems were just blisters, which I have dealt with before. I even brought something to clean the areas and pop the blisters if necessary.

I didn't realize it at the time, but my feet were wet. I was sweating, and spectators and volunteers were pouring water on and spraying the athletes down with water in certain parts of the course. My feet were developing blisters because they were wet, and the repetitive contact with the ground was heating up my feet. Plus, without doing a lot of training miles, the skin on my feet simply wasn't tough enough to handle all the mileage.

I had the opportunity to access my Run Special Needs Bag at mile ten, but I passed because I didn't want to stop so early in the marathon. I would have another opportunity to pick it up on my final loop at mile nineteen. I figured that was a better time to access the bag, which was only available to athletes once. If I went into the bag at mile ten, I couldn't access it again at mile nineteen. There was nutrition I placed into the bag that I would need more during my third loop than during my second loop and didn't want to carry it.

That was probably a mistake because inside my Run Special Needs Bag was a pair of dry socks.

After passing the opportunity to access my Run Special Needs Bag at mile ten, I sat down at the next Aid Station for a few minutes. When I stood back up, my feet hurt like hell. I was eleven miles into the 26.2-mile route. I had heard about runners getting stress fractures in the small bones in their feet after endurance events, and I wondered if I had done just that. Every step hurt, but the pain was manageable. I was finishing the IRONMAN event no matter what.

I continued passing the time and the miles talking with other athletes, spectators, and volunteers. The sun set during my first loop of the marathon course, and it was motivating to see the excitement even late into the night. Part of the course was a tree-covered path lit up with Christmas lights. There were neon lights, spectators in costumes, and music playing throughout the course. The local community in The Woodlands really embraced the event. It was exciting to be part of it all, even if I was in some pain.

I walked the last two miles of my second loop with two athletes finishing their third and final loop. They veered off at the appropriate place toward the finish line, and I had to keep going. I was a little disappointed to still have another nine miles to go, which would take over two more hours to complete.

There were still athletes on the course late into the night, and many were walking. I guess the heat and the long day slowed many athletes down. Walking all or a portion of the marathon course was more common than I thought it would be. I met a lot of athletes while we walked and talked. I met some athletes, like me, who were doing their first IRONMAN triathlon while others had done more than a dozen.

I was doing everything I could to take my mind off my feet. Spending time with other athletes helped the miles and time pass.

As I started my third loop, I knew the area to access my Special Needs Bag was only about a mile away. I couldn't wait to get there. As I crested a bridge, I could see the area in the distance. It was in a well-lit park where the swim start was earlier in the day, and I could see the volunteers organizing the remaining bags and scrambling to get bags to athletes. Somehow, I picked up my pace, knowing there was something I put into my bag to help me.

As I approached the Special Needs Bag area, I called out my athlete number, and a volunteer came running with my bag. I knew my feet were swollen, and it would be painful to stand back up if I sat down, but I had to do something. My left foot was much worse than my right.

*If I take my shoes off, will it hurt more than it does now?* I thought. *Will I be able to put my shoes back on?*

*Screw it, take off the shoe and fix what I can. I have time. The pain is temporary. It will be gone in a few days.*

For the second time during the marathon, I sat down. I found a bench under a park light. I had to try to mitigate my foot pain as much as possible. I was going to regret it, but my plan was to pop the blisters, change into dry socks, get up, and finish.

It felt good to get the shoes off. It didn't feel great, though. My feet throbbed. It was just a different pain, but a different pain was welcome.

As I sat there, several athletes passed by and encouraged me to get back up and finish. We were on the same page, but I had some work to do first. At no point was quitting an option. I glanced at my triathlon plan on the laminated card and knew I had extra time to address my foot issues.

After peeling off my right sock, I saw that all the blisters on my right foot had already popped. I then peeled off my left sock. I was stunned to see no blisters there, but what had happened was much worse. The skin on half the bottom of my foot was torn away and rolled up under the base of my toes. I tried unrolling it, but it was stuck, and I didn't have enough time or the tools to try and fix it. The exposed raw foot where the missing skin used to be was being burned with each step from the friction of walking with wet socks and shoes.

I also noticed that three toenails on my left foot, starting from the big toe, were ready to fall off.

I knew all the pain was temporary, and I was enjoying the experience because it was something out of the ordinary. I volunteered for this and was having fun. (Really!)

My feet were swollen and sore to the touch, but I was only eight miles away from finishing the IRONMAN event. The total distance of an IRONMAN triathlon is 140.6 miles, and I had completed thousands of training miles and spent almost three years preparing. I only had eight miles left to finish my journey. At my current pace, that would take about two hours.

I put on dry socks, squeezed my feet back into my shoes, and stood up. The burning sensation in my feet was immediate. I put one foot in front of the other and kept moving—the thought of not finishing never crossed my mind.

I counted down the miles and knew I still had plenty of time to finish before the seventeen-hour time limit. I was hurrying more to get off my feet than I was to save time.

There were lots of athletes still walking out on the course. The heat was getting to many of them. I actually passed athletes. It had been dark for several hours already, and the night was getting eerily intense.

The last mile was the worst. The course came close to the finish line but then veered off another half mile before coming back to the finish. I could hear the excitement from the finish line and the announcer before turning away again to do the last half-mile out and back portion to finish the last mile.

## THE FINISH

The IRONMAN triathlon finish includes bright lights, loud music, and a long red carpet. Typically, an athlete can see the finish and all the lights from a distance. The Woodlands has a strange finish because it's in an entertainment district with bars and restaurants lining the streets. There's normally a lot of people, music, and activity on a Saturday night anyway, and this night was no different. There's also not a long straight road leading up to the finish. I knew I was getting close because the road was sectioned off with guard rails, creating a finishing chute, and only athletes were allowed inside the chute. I could hear the finish line long before seeing it. It wasn't until I was almost on top of the finish that I could actually see it. The finishing chute made a few quick turns around a building, and I saw the finish line about fifty yards in front of me. I high-fived a lot of the spectators along the barriers of the finishing chute and leisurely walked up to the finish line. I was in no hurry to let the moment pass.

As I walked under the IRONMAN banner at the finish line, I couldn't see much because of all the bright lights pointed in my direction, but I heard the announcer say the famous line . . .

*"Chris Bystriansky, YOU ARE AN IRONMAN!"*

I finished the marathon in seven hours and twenty-three minutes, and my total time was sixteen hours and sixteen minutes, well within the seventeen-hour time limit. I stayed on my plan all day and finished just three minutes and sixteen seconds ahead of my projected finish time (a table showing time splits for each IRONMAN triathlon is provided after the Conclusion).

A volunteer put an IRONMAN triathlon finisher medal around my neck and handed me a hat and T-shirt. As relieved and happy as I was, I just wanted to get off my feet. Unfortunately, I was in such a hurry to get off my feet that I made a major rookie mistake. I failed to get my picture in front of the IRONMAN triathlon finisher backdrop.

A few friends found me, and we walked a short distance to the area to pick up my Morning Bag and get some water. We found a table with chairs and sat down. It was midnight.

## AFTER THE FINISH

I sat there for about ten minutes talking with my friends and then decided it was time to go back to the hotel, which was just a short distance. I walked past the finishing chute and watched a few more athletes cross the finish line. It was an electric atmosphere—a big party cheering people on as they completed something remarkable. I wanted to stay longer and cheer for athletes as they finished, but I had to get off my feet.

I went to my hotel room, changed my clothes, and then had to pick up my bike and T1 and T2 bags by 1:00 a.m. Everything was located in the Transition area, about a quarter mile away. I decided to drive there because there was no way I was walking that extra mileage to the Transition area and then back to the hotel. It was 1:45 before I was back in my hotel room with my bike and all my gear.

I showered, sat in a chair with my feet in a bucket of ice, and watched TV until 4:00 a.m. It was a long day, but I was too wound up to sleep earlier.

## RECOVERY

The next morning, I slept in until 8:00 a.m. I was sore and gently walked around the hotel lobby talking with friends and other athletes. My family met me there for breakfast and helped me get packed up. There was still some excitement in the area, and it was great for my wife and kids to experience that.

In the days following, my feet got worse. Maybe I was just coming down from the high of the event, and I couldn't feel the extent of the pain sooner. I couldn't even walk on them later in the week. I hobbled around my house before finally deciding to use crutches. I had blisters on the tips of my toes, and I lost three toenails on my left foot. I put cream on the bottoms of my feet to ease the burning pain.

I went to see a sports medicine doctor specializing in foot injuries. I was concerned about stress fractures. I thought I broke the bones in my left foot. I needed to heal quickly because I had another IRONMAN triathlon scheduled in less than six weeks.

The doctor came in and looked.

"What did you do to your feet?" he asked.

"IRONMAN," I said.

"Did you train at all, or did you just show up?"

I agree my feet didn't look like I had trained much, which was actually the case. I hadn't put a lot of miles on my feet in over three months. Without the mileage leading up to the event, my feet were unprepared for the beating they took.

I explained that I tore the meniscus in my left knee in July, and my mileage had been cut way down in recent months, leaving my feet unprepared for the triathlon. Plus, I told him it was hot and my feet were wet, which led to the blisters.

He just looked at my feet without saying much. He appeared agitated with me for some reason.

My feet were really swollen.

I had X-rays, which came back negative for broken bones, but the doctor explained that stress fractures might be too small to show up on X-rays.

*Perfect!* I thought.

"How long will those take to heal?" I asked.

"It depends."

Half the skin on my left foot had rolled up to the base of my toes. The doctor unrolled the skin and cut it off, revealing more tender and bruised tissue underneath.

The official diagnosis was second-degree burns caused by the heat and friction on my feet during the IRONMAN event.

He gave me a prescription for medicated cream, put my left foot into a small boot, and told me to come back in a week.

The foot got somewhat better over the next week, and I returned to see him without the boot or the crutches.

While my right foot was almost back to normal, my left foot was still swollen and tender to the touch. He advised me to stay off my feet as much as possible for another few weeks.

"I have another IRONMAN event in four weeks," I said.

"Maybe," he responded. "You may want to consider skipping it."

I didn't care for his pessimistic outlook. "I don't think so."

There was no more conversation until we were outside the exam room.

"When are you going to stop doing crazy things?" he asked.

"Being cooped up in an office all day and not experiencing life is crazy," I said. "Besides, I'd rather be a participant in life and not just a spectator."

He didn't care for my answer. He shook his head and walked away.

The feeling was mutual.

I was on crutches for almost two weeks because of my left foot, and it took a month for the skin to heal. Less than three weeks after leaving the doctor's office, I was in Arizona for my next IRONMAN triathlon.

# 11

# TRIATHLON #2—
# IRONMAN ARIZONA

As soon as I could, I got back into the pool and on the bike to prepare. I didn't get much training done during the six weeks between IRONMAN events because my left foot was torn up. I needed it to heal, so I stayed off it. I relaxed for three weeks, trained for two weeks, and then jumped on a plane for Arizona. The lack of training didn't matter, though. I had been down this road before and learned how to make it work.

I was so relaxed. It must have been a mix of confidence or burnout from training. I didn't even have my suitcase packed with all the required gear until the night before my morning flight.

*Shouldn't I be more concerned?* I thought.

Any fear or trepidation I had in the days and weeks leading up to the first IRONMAN triathlon was nonexistent before the second one. Despite the foot issue, torn meniscus, and two replaced hips, I knew everything was going to be okay.

Going to Arizona felt like a business trip to me—business that I had to take care of. There was no sense of closure for me after finishing the first IRONMAN event. I heard stories about and even witnessed people finishing the triathlon and becoming so overwhelmed with emotion that they broke down in tears. That's a perfectly appropriate reaction because it's a long and difficult journey to get to the finish line. I feel like I missed that for some reason.

Somewhere along the line, possibly after all the cancellations and rescheduling set up the IRONMAN events only six weeks apart, my original goal of finishing one IRONMAN triathlon was not big enough. Originally, the events were scheduled six months apart. When that was the schedule, my goal was to finish the first one and maybe not even go to the second one. When they were rescheduled to be only six weeks apart, it triggered something inside me. I began thinking that I was fortunate to have the opportunity to do two so close to each other. I felt an internal drive and a sense of obligation to finish both. I no longer had the goal of finishing one IRONMAN triathlon. I had a mission to finish two.

That is why I didn't have a sense of closure or overwhelming joy after my first IRONMAN triathlon finish. I certainly felt a sense of accomplishment and was pleased with my achievement but knew I was only halfway done.

When you have a goal, it's dependent on other circumstances. It's subject to disruption. But when you have a mission, it's not negotiable, and anything less than success is not an option. There's a much different mindset between the two. Things can get in the way of a goal, but nothing can stop you from completing a mission because a mission has a deeper sense of purpose.

It's certainly better to set goals than not to do anything and coast through life. A goal is a nice thing to accomplish. You can negotiate with a goal because it wraps around your lifestyle and is secondary to it. With a goal, obstacles need to be overcome.

A mission is not flexible. When you have a mission, it becomes your central focus. Your life wraps around the mission, and your lifestyle is secondary to the mission. With a mission, obstacles don't exist because you'll go right past whatever excuses stand between you and accomplishing your mission.

A goal is something nice or beneficial to accomplish. A mission is something that must be accomplished. That's the difference between having a goal and having a mission.

That's why I wasn't concerned. I was on a mission. No obstacle mattered. I found everything to be easier and with less uncertainty. I was focused only on the finish line. My foot, knee, hips, weather conditions, strange environment, and lack of training were all irrelevant. My plan was to ignore the issues I could, mitigate the rest, and get to the finish line.

## NOVEMBER 2021

This was a full-size IRONMAN event with over 2,000 athletes. It was evident as soon as I saw all the vendors and support in the IRONMAN Village and the size of the Transition area. The IRONMAN Village and the Transition area were set up in Tempe Beach Park along the lakefront. I didn't see any beach, though, and I wasn't sure why there would be a beach there anyway. Regardless, the park was pretty large, and the event seemed back to normal following the virus. I looked forward to the crowd and the energy of triathlon day.

## TIME AND STRATEGY

The time limit for this IRONMAN triathlon was sixteen hours and forty minutes. That seemed like a strange cutoff time, but it may have had to do with permitting or other local requirements. The time limit for the IRONMAN event in Texas was seventeen hours. The shorter time limit in Arizona meant I had less margin for error. My goal, again, was to finish within the time limits. I had to be fast enough in the water and on the bike to make up for a slower marathon time.

I used the same laminated card with my projected split times for each segment from the last IRONMAN event. It worked so well six weeks earlier that I was going to use it again. The card showed my projected times, so if I was slower than expected on an earlier segment, I would need to increase my pace going forward.

I also would wear two watches again. With the shorter time cutoff, I knew I would be cutting it very close, so knowing my total time (on one watch) and my pacing (on another watch) was critical.

## TRANSPORTATION AND LODGING

I stayed at the AC Hotel Phoenix Tempe because it was the closest hotel to the start, finish, and Transition area. It's only about a quarter mile away. I booked ten months in advance to ensure I had a room reserved there because, logistically, it was the easiest place to stay. I could walk back and forth to the IRONMAN Village and Transition area rather than having to drive and find a place to park each time. That was important to me during the morning and evening of the event.

The triathlon was on a Sunday, and I was uncertain how many days early I would arrive before the event and how long I would stay after. Although the hotel required full nonrefundable prepayment at the time of booking, I reserved a room from the Wednesday before the event until the Tuesday following the event.

I started the reservation on Wednesday rather than Thursday because I didn't know how early I would need to arrive. Ten months before the event, I was still uncertain if I would be driving or flying to Arizona. If I were driving the eighteen hours from Houston to Arizona, I certainly would have wanted to arrive a day or two earlier than normal to give my body time to recover from the long drive.

I decided to fly rather than drive. I still arrived on Wednesday because I scheduled business meetings with contacts in the area on Thursday and Friday. It also gave me more time to acclimate to the climate and surroundings.

In hindsight, that was probably one day too early. I didn't have much preparation left to do with my gear, and although I took care of some business, I found myself sitting around more than I liked.

After the IRONMAN triathlon, I flew home late Monday afternoon even though the hotel reservation was through Tuesday. I couldn't change the reservation to get my money back for the extra hotel night, but I was ready to get home. Again, when I booked the hotel earlier in the year, there was a possibility of me driving, and I didn't want to start the long drive home the day immediately after the event because I didn't know how sore I would be.

I also didn't realize the hotel allowed pets on certain floors, and there were dogs barking on my floor. If you stay there, or any hotel, I suggest checking their policies and requesting a room on a floor with no pets. There were a couple of nights when dogs were barking late at night.

The hotel was surrounded by condos and office buildings. I had a rental car, so I was able to get to restaurants and grocery stores for last-minute supplies. Although the hotel was convenient for the event, there wasn't much else close to the hotel.

## BIKE TRANSPORTATION

A triathlon bike transport company shipped my bike. It cost about $400, but they shipped my bike fully assembled except for the pedals, which was a big benefit. I wasn't interested in disassembling my bike myself, packing it into a special bike case, and then trying to put it back together myself to the exact same specs it was previously. Having my bike show up with the exact same specs as during my training was worth the cost. Plus, there was a significant convenience factor. All I had to do was remove the pedals and drop my bike off at a designated bike shop in the Houston area. I could then pick it up in the Transition area three days before the IRONMAN event. The bike transport company even put the pedals back on for me. I aired up the tires and was ready to go.

After the triathlon, all I had to do was take my bike back to the bike transport tent, which was conveniently located next to the Transition area and the bike compound. They would then deliver it back to the local bike shop in the Houston area, where I could pick it up about a week later.

The only downside was how early I had to drop my bike off at the bike shop in Houston, so my bike could be transported to Arizona. I dropped it off eleven days before the IRONMAN event. Without my bike for that long, I missed a few training sessions.

## TEMPE, ARIZONA

The environment was dry and dusty. I noticed a thin layer of dust on everything. There was no noticeable humidity, which was unusual for me, being from the Houston area where humidity ranges between 50 and 80 percent most of the year. The starting elevation in Tempe was only about 1,000 feet, so elevation didn't cause any breathing difficulty, but the dry and dusty air had an impact. There's a big difference between that and breathing in humid air. When humidity is lower, I feel like it's slightly more difficult to breathe.

Humid air holds less oxygen than dry air, but I still find it easier to breathe when the humidity is high. That may be because the humidity lubricates lungs and air passages, whereas dry air may irritate the air passages. It's the same concept as using humidifiers in a home.

I spent a lot of time walking back and forth between the hotel and the Triathlon Village to shop at all the vendors, check in for the event, and attend the Athlete Briefing, along with a host of other events. While spending so much time outside, I had to be careful to stay hydrated.

When it's hot and humid, I sweat, so it's easy to notice liquid leaving my body. I sweat, so therefore I must drink. It's simple. In a dry climate, however, there's little to no sweat, but the body is still losing moisture into the air. Dehydration can sneak up on you. I was constantly drinking to ensure I stayed hydrated. One of the last things anyone wants in an IRONMAN triathlon is to start dehydrated because there's no way to catch up on hydration on event day.

# T MINUS TWO DAYS

## WARM-UP BIKE RIDE

Two days before the IRONMAN triathlon, I participated in a group warm-up ride. The purpose of the ride wasn't to train but to ensure your bike was working properly and to get a feel for the course. The bike route was three loops of an out-and-back course that started at Tempe Beach Park at the Transition area and climbed over the nineteen-mile stretch northeast into the surrounding foothills.

TriDot®, a leading triathlon coaching platform and podcast, organized the warm-up ride. About forty riders met at the farthest point of the route. I drove with a friend out to the start. After announcements and introductions, the group rode downhill toward town about ten miles before turning around and climbing back to finish the warm-up ride.

The route was notorious for road debris, and flat tires were common. Sure enough, I experienced a flat tire about five miles from the finish. I stopped with some friends to fix the tire. I pulled a six-inch-long metal wire, a little thicker than a hair, from the tire. I finished the ride without another incident.

## ATHLETE CHECK-IN

I officially checked in for the event at Triathlon Village after the morning warm-up ride. The Triathlon Village was the central location for the event. It included many vendor tents, official trailers, and the Transition area, including the bike compound. I picked up my timing ankle bracelet, number bib, wristband, and some swag items. I also picked up the five gear bags I would use throughout the day.

There is not supposed to be any check-in on the day of the event or the day before the event. I imagine extenuating circumstances could call for an exception to that policy once in a while, but I didn't have any of those, so I checked in two days before the event.

# T MINUS ONE DAY

## BIKE REPAIR

Since the warm-up bike ride was still two days before the event, and bikes were not to be checked in until the following day, I kept my bike overnight in my hotel room. The next morning, I checked the tires again and had another flat.

I ride a Quintana Roo triathlon bike, and one of the great things about Quintana Roo is that they often have tents at the Triathlon Village to promote their bikes and other products. What they also have are mechanics who service Quintana Roo bikes. So, if you have one of their bikes and you take it to their tent, they'll take care of you. The alternative is to use third-party mechanics, which often come with long lines and high costs. I dropped my bike off at the Quintana Roo tent as soon as it opened, explained the problem, and had my bike back in an hour. I had no further bike problems, and my bike was perfect.

## PRACTICE SWIM

As is tradition, there is a practice swim the day before the IRONMAN event. The swim was set up similar to the start of the actual swim with an announcer, music, spectators, and lots of athletes. The atmosphere is already pretty electric the day before the triathlon, and it all starts with the practice swim because this is the first time most athletes are in the same place at about the same time.

The practice swim was in the same lake as the actual event swim. It was close to my hotel, less than a five-minute walk. Even with the close proximity, I got there toward the end of the window of time to get in the water because I was busy addressing my bike issue earlier.

It was late morning with temps at just sixty degrees. There was a slight breeze, and the sun was shining. Thousands of people, including athletes and spectators, filled the greenspace that separated the lakefront from the high-rise office buildings and condos. I found a nice shady spot to put my things down in a less crowded area. It was like an outdoor festival with music and people everywhere. From my vantage point uphill from the lake, I could see hundreds of athletes already in the water, making their way around the short swim course. The swim course was shaped like a big rectangle, laid out in the water with large pyramid-shaped red inflatable buoys. Athletes entered the water and then swam clockwise around the course.

As I watched the athletes in the water, I carefully put on my wetsuit, which took about ten minutes. The wetsuits tear easily, and it's advised to put them on slowly to reduce the risk of tearing the material. It also took time to ensure the wetsuit was in the right position. It's tight, no doubt about it, and it takes time to work it into the correct position. For example, if the shoulder in the wetsuit is not in the correct place on your body when you put it on, it can negatively impact the swim because it makes it more difficult to move the arm and shoulder properly and, therefore, make an efficient swim stroke.

Even after taking ten minutes to put on my wetsuit and ankle timing bracelet, there was still a long line of athletes waiting to get into the water. I waited about ten minutes. As I stood in line, athletes getting out of the water were walking past me in the opposite direction. Some of them commented that the water was really cold. Some said it was refreshing. Some just looked miserable. I knew the water would be cold, so I prepared for it.

• • •

After growing up in the cold Midwest and playing hockey outside all winter, I no longer enjoyed being in the cold as I got older. But this being an IRONMAN triathlon, it didn't matter what the water temperature was. It was just one of those things to overcome.

As I mentioned earlier, the pool complex I used back in the Houston area has two outdoor pools. One of the pools is sometimes heated during the winter, and the other pool is not heated at all. My standard process through each winter was jumping into the cold pool and then hurrying over to the heated pool to start my workouts. It has become more common for overnight temps to drop into the 30's and 40's so the water was pretty cold throughout the winter.

I hated doing that, especially in the early mornings. I did it, though, to prepare myself for this moment in Arizona. And frankly, because it was a little crazy, deep down, there was something appealing about it. Cold plunges take some discipline, and I felt that if I could do this, I could tackle other difficult tasks.

• • •

As my turn approached to begin the practice swim, I put on my swim cap and goggles and walked down the ramp toward the water. I first felt the sting of the cold water on my feet. I continued walking forward, following about twenty feet behind the athlete in front of me. The water came up over my knees and then my waist before I finally dove forward into the water. My hands, neck, and face all felt the cold. The sense of shock, common in open water swims, hit me quickly, and I struggled to catch my breath for a few strokes.

The rest of the swim was uneventful. It was only about 500 meters, which took around ten minutes. When I reached the exit and started walking up the ramp, I noticed the line of athletes to get into the water was still long. I took my wetsuit off carefully, got my stuff together, and walked back to my hotel. I still had a lot to do that day.

## MARATHON ROUTE

After lunch, I took my bike for a short ride to check out the tires and ensure they were alright. The roads in the area had a lot of traffic, so I rode around the marathon route, which was mostly on a path and sidewalks. The marathon route was a nine-mile loop, which was to be covered three times during the triathlon.

It was a great way to see the route and get familiar with the settings before the event. There were a few areas of the route where athletes would go out and come back on the same path. Looking at the course map, it was hard to determine the exact route, so I lost the route a few different times and took some time to figure it out. Part of the marathon route was on a dirt path along the lake. I didn't want to ride my bike on the soft powdering dirt, so I followed a nearby concrete path.

It was a good idea to get familiar with the route, particularly when I wasn't tired like I would be at the back end of the triathlon the next day. I noted the features and where I would need extra effort or focus on certain areas of the route. I saw where all the Aid Stations and turnarounds were being set up. I also noticed where the elevation changes were. There were some ramps to different levels of the path early in the route, about mile two, and then there was a hill toward the back of the route, about mile six.

## GEAR BAGS

By mid-afternoon, I was back in my hotel room. I had another lunch and sat down to rest and watch some TV. My bike and Transition 1 (T1) and Transition 2 (T2) gear bags were to be dropped off later in the afternoon. But it was time to relax. I laid out the empty bags on the bed. The T1 bag was to be filled with the items I needed to transition from the swim to the bike segments. The T2 bag was to be filled with the items I needed to transition from the bike to the marathon segments.

I must have zoned out for a while because the next thing I knew, I looked at my watch and realized I had less than an hour to get my gear bags packed and take them and my bike to the Transition area. It was late afternoon the day before the event. I have no idea what the consequence would have been, if any, had I been late, but I didn't want to find out.

I needed to get my T1 and T2 bags packed quickly. The other bags, including the Bike Special Needs, Run Special Needs, and Morning bags, could wait because they didn't have to be dropped off until the next morning. I pulled out the envelope I had received at Athlete Check-In and grabbed the stickers with my athlete number. The stickers were to be placed on each bag and bike so everyone, including athletes and volunteers, could identify the bags and bikes. I was warned that the bags would be left outside overnight and that any dew could make the stickers fall off, so I put bright pink duct tape on my bags and wrote my athlete number on the tape. That would be a nightmare for everyone if the standard-issued stickers came off the transition bags. No one would be able to find their stuff because all the bags looked the same.

I had a checklist of what to pack in each bag and quickly filled them up. I made the checklist while preparing for my first IRONMAN triathlon. The difference, though, was at the first IRONMAN event, I went through the list at least five times and packed, unpacked, and repacked the bags over several days to ensure I wasn't missing anything. This time around, at the second IRONMAN triathlon, I went down the list and shoved the items in the appropriate bags less than an hour before they needed to be dropped off. The checklist even had a lot of items crossed off because I didn't use them the first time around. After they were packed, I put the T1 and T2 bags by the door.

Next, I quickly checked all the gear on my bike to ensure I had the tools needed. I packed my T1 and T2 bags, made sure my bike was ready, and walked to the Transition area in less than forty-five minutes. That same prep was spread out over several days for my first IRONMAN event.

## TRANSITION AREA

By the time I arrived at the Transition area, there were thousands of bags there, all laid out in numerical order. The blue T1 bags were in one area, and the red T2 bags were in a different area. I handed my bags to the volunteers, who then arranged them in their appropriate places.

The bags for the different transitions were separated and staged in areas that made it efficient for the athletes. When exiting the swim segment, athletes would enter the Transition area from the east side, so the T1 bags were placed near the east park entrance. When finishing the bike segment, athletes would ride into the park from the south, so the T2 bags were placed close to the south entrance. A large tent was set up nearby for athletes to change clothes if they desired. It was an efficient process flow into and out of Transition.

After dropping off my T1 and T2 bags, I took my bike into the bike compound. Since I was there pretty late in the afternoon, there were already thousands of bikes staged on the bike racks, all organized numerically. The bike compound was fenced off, and there were only two ways in and out, which had a heavy volunteer presence. With all the value of the bikes sitting there overnight, it made sense that they didn't want the bikes to leave the compound with the wrong person.

Later that night, I packed my Bike Special Needs bag with some extra nutrition, spare inner tubes, and $CO_2$ cartridges in the event I had to use the ones I was carrying with me on my bike. I'd be able to pick up the bag one time on either lap two or lap three of the ride. I also packed my T2 bag with nutrition and, of course, some extra socks in case my feet were wet. I'd be able to pick up the bag one time on either lap two or lap three of the marathon.

## SLEEP

I went to sleep each night at about 9:00 p.m. and woke up at about 4:00 a.m. to stay on a consistent schedule. I slept great each night I was there except for the night before the event. I again went to sleep at about 9:00 p.m. and, rather than sleep through the night, I woke up at some point overnight. There was no danger of oversleeping because I had two alarms set and a wake-up call scheduled.

Now, one thing about me is that I'm usually a pretty good sleeper, and if I wake up overnight, I do my best not to look at a clock to find out what time it is. If I look at a clock, it's almost guaranteed I won't fall back asleep. So, my practice at home was to avoid looking at the time and try to fall back asleep. Only after a long time of rolling around in bed and failing to fall back asleep will I check the time and likely get up at that point.

I eventually fell back asleep, but I knew I was awake for a while. When the alarms sounded, I was not rested and knew I didn't get a decent night's sleep. I don't know exactly but based on how I felt, I estimate I only got about four or five hours of broken sleep.

You know what, though? I didn't care. I had actually trained a few times with little sleep just to prepare for that scenario. One time, I slept about three hours and woke up overnight. I couldn't fall back asleep, so I got up and went to the pool. It was my earliest swim ever, and I ended up swimming 4,000 meters before 6:00 a.m., which is the IRONMAN triathlon distance. I also did the 4x4x48 (four miles every four hours for forty-eight hours as described above) earlier in 2021. I did many of the miles on very little sleep, which is one of the elements of the challenge. That kind of training earlier in the year helped me not care about lack of sleep.

Those were some of my hardest and most unreasonable training sessions. They helped me grow mentally and physically. I knew I could finish this IRONMAN event, regardless of my sleep results.

# T MINUS ZERO DAYS - IT'S TRIATHLON DAY!

## MORNING

When I got out of bed at 4:00 a.m., I lounged around the hotel room. I turned the TV on, ate breakfast, and packed up a few final items. I was way too relaxed, even by my standards, and there was no sense of urgency. I was running late but didn't care. Everything was going to be fine. I left the hotel room thirty minutes later than I wanted, which meant I was in danger of not being allowed into the Transition area. It closes a set amount of time before the scheduled start time.

Athletes want to get into the Transition area, particularly the bike compound, on the morning of the triathlon to fill up their bike tires with air and fill up their water bottles, which they leave on their bikes and make any last-minute changes to their T1 and T2 bags. Plus, the Transition area is where the Special Needs and Morning bags were to be dropped off.

I probably walked the path from the hotel to the Transition area at least twenty times throughout the days of the event. Most athletes were leaving the Transition area when I arrived. I dropped off my Special Needs bag and then went to my bike to fill up my water bottles and my tires.

Announcements were blaring that Transition was closing, and all athletes were to make their way to the swim start, about a quarter mile away.

I was still at my bike. There were very few other athletes around, and volunteers were walking through the bike compound, ushering athletes out.

What was I to do?

No worries. I didn't feel late. I was just on *my* time schedule.

I took off everything except my swim shorts and carefully put my wetsuit halfway on, up to my waist. I then put on my ankle timing bracelet. I stuffed all my clothes, glasses, room key, and phone into my Morning bag and walked it over to the designated drop-off zone.

It was still dark outside and cool, about fifty degrees. The wetsuits can get hot, so I was comfortable walking with it halfway up. It was about 6:40 a.m., and given the number of athletes, I figured I still had about thirty minutes before getting into the water.

There were still a lot of people, including athletes and spectators, walking on the path to the swim start. It was a long column of people, shoulder to shoulder. I was toward the back of the column and knew I didn't want to start near the back of the group because it would have taken a long time to even get into the water. When the path widened, I was able to work my way up through the crowd and find the volunteer holding up a sign with my swim speed. I wanted to self-seed myself into the group that anticipated finishing the swim between 1:20 and 1:30. I worked my way into that general area.

## TEN MINUTES TO GO

The column of people narrowed again to about twelve feet wide, and only athletes were allowed to continue on the path. Spectators lined the barricades along the left side of the path, and the lake, separated by a three-foot-high concrete wall, was on the right side of the path.

Everyone else had their wetsuits fully on. I still only had mine partially on. I was warm, being in the middle of the group of athletes. I heard other athletes comment on how hot they were. The last thing I wanted was to get hot and then jump into the cold water.

It was barely light outside, but there were already athletes in the water. Even though they started ten or twenty minutes before me, it didn't impact my time. Each athlete had the full sixteen hours and forty minutes, which started when their ankle timing bracelet crossed the start line before getting into the water.

I started to pull up the remainder of my wetsuit. It was hard to finish putting it on standing so close to other athletes. There's a lot of wiggling and stretching when putting on a wetsuit, and I did my best not to hit anyone accidentally.

Once I had the wetsuit in the proper placement around my arms and shoulders, I reached behind to zip up the back, but another athlete standing behind me kindly finished zipping it up for me.

## FIVE MINUTES TO GO

I inched forward with the group every few seconds. I could finally see the start about ten feet in front of me. There was an inflatable arched banner that athletes went under, and I could see the announcer getting the crowd worked up. Again, there were five chutes for athletes to enter and then wait their turn. About every five seconds, there was a loud beep, and that group of five athletes entered the water.

With about a minute to go, I knew which chute I was going into. The swim route called for swimmers to enter the water and make an immediate right turn, swim across the narrow lake about a hundred meters, and then make another right to swim the long back straightaway. Since I could see the first few turns, I noticed where swimmers were getting bunched up. I watched and picked my anticipated swim line to ensure I would not get bunched up with the other swimmers at the first few turns.

I put on my swim cap and goggles and waited. A minute later, I was standing at the front in my chute. A volunteer told me good luck, and then I heard the loud beep.

It was go-time.

## SWIM

I walked down the ramp, and when the water was waist-deep, I dove in to start swimming. The cold water hitting my face was a shock. I took a few deep breaths to calm down and settled into a smooth rhythm.

I swam wide on the first few turns because athletes can get a little excited and swim fast at the start. There's a lot of bumping around turns early in a swim, and I wanted no part of that. I stayed on the line I picked out earlier and made it to the long back stretch without incident.

My plan was to start slow and finish slow. I wanted to conserve as much energy as possible for the later segments. The swim is the shortest segment in an IRONMAN triathlon, and an incredible effort in the water simply won't save much time. The difference between a moderate, energy-conserving swim and an aggressive fast swim may only be ten to twenty minutes. To me, that time savings wasn't worth the risk of burning out too early.

I actually enjoyed the swim. Within five minutes, I didn't notice the cold anymore. We had to swim under a few bridges, which were lined with spectators. I avoided the big concrete pillars holding up the bridges and did my best to wave at the spectators.

The weather was overcast, windy, and about fifty degrees. The water was slightly choppy from the wind, making the buoys a little difficult to see. I don't think there were enough buoys. It seemed like a long distance between them. Still, I sighted well, and I was able to stay online throughout the swim. Each time I passed a buoy, it was about ten feet to my right, which seemed about perfect. There were a few left turns toward the end, and the buoys were about ten feet to my left. It was a good swim.

I had a lot of space. After the first few turns, the swim didn't feel congested until the last few tight turns near the end. With each breath I took, I looked at the shoreline and occasionally looked forward to check my direction. I stayed relaxed the entire time in the water. As with many of my training swims, I must have zoned out, thinking about other things, because the time passed by quickly.

There were boats and kayaks with officials, lifeguards, and volunteers along the swim route. As before, athletes could take a break by holding onto one of the boats or kayaks as long as they didn't push off when they restarted their swim. I suppose there would have been time penalties if any athletes had pushed off. I didn't stop during the swim. I'm a fairly strong swimmer and never felt the need.

Just over one hour and twenty-five minutes after getting into the water, I walked up the finishing ramp to get out. My IRONMAN triathlon swim was over.

## TRANSITION ONE

The swim finished where the practice swim was held the day before. It was on the same side of the lake but farther east than the swim start. It was close to my hotel but a quarter mile away from the Transition area. Many athletes lightly jogged from the swim finish to the Transition area. I walked. I had plenty of time. Volunteers were available to help athletes quickly strip off their wetsuits, but I passed on the help. I slowly took the top of my wetsuit off while I walked. I high-fived a few spectators who lined the barricades and continued onward.

I followed the barriers, which snaked through to the entrance to the Transition. A volunteer asked for my athlete number. I looked down at my wristband, which conveniently included my number. I called out my number, which was relayed to other volunteers, and someone came running with my T1 bag.

There was a big changing tent available, but I changed outside, along with many other athletes. About half of the hundreds of athletes around me were in a rush, but I was totally relaxed. Many athletes do the entire event in the same shorts or a onesie triathlon suit. That wasn't me. I wanted clean, dry clothes on. I dumped the contents of my T1 bag on the ground and then pulled off the rest of my wetsuit. I wrapped a towel around my waist and changed into standard cycling shorts underneath.

I brushed my teeth, ate, drank, used the porta-john, chatted with spectators and volunteers, dropped off my T1 bag with the volunteers, and then went to the bike compound to claim my bike.

It was a big area and I was forced to take a long path, which was not the most direct, to my bike. It took a while just to get to my bike. Although I was moving faster than the T1 in my first IRONMAN event, my time was longer. There was simply a lot of distance to cover, which increased my time. Over twenty-three minutes after leaving the water, I was through Transition and on my bike.

## BIKE

The bike segment was three loops of an out-and-back route—nineteen miles out and nineteen miles back. There were two sections to the route. The first section, about eight miles, was through main city streets and neighborhoods. It was a slight incline going out with a few flat portions and into the wind or crosswind. The second section, about eleven miles, was on the Beeline Highway, which headed northeast, up into the foothills. This second section was a little steeper, between a 2 and 4 percent grade, and windier than the first section. The northbound side of the Beeline Highway was closed to traffic and open only to riders and official vehicles.

The Beeline Highway section was pretty barren with no protection from the wind. It was a desert. The route was uphill going out, and the wind was either directly at me or slightly from the left as the route curved. It was blowing between 10 and 15 miles per hour. The route became steeper and the wind more intense toward the farthest point of the route.

On my first loop, I focused on maintaining a steady pace and getting enough food and hydration. I started strong but slowed significantly on the Beeline Highway segment. The wind and slight incline took their toll. Once I reached the turnaround point at the farthest part of the route, it was mostly downhill coming back, and I figured I could make up some time. The problem I found was that the road was very bumpy, and the faster I rode, the more difficult it was to control my bike. I guess this type of bumpy road texture was required due to the heat in the summer. When roads are bumpy, bike tires are not in constant contact with the road, and bikes are harder to control.

If the rough road wasn't enough, about every fifty yards, there was a gap in the pavement. Again, it was probably designed that way to allow the concrete room to expand in the summer heat. Every time I rode over a gap, there was a big jolt to the bike. My bike was constantly vibrating, and I was gripping my bars tight just to hang on.

The wind was at my back and slightly over my right shoulder, but there were times with strong crosswind gusts. The faster I rode, the less control I had. Since I was fighting to maintain control over my bike, I slowed my pace to make it through the first loop safely. I should have been able to come down the hill around 30 miles per hour but came down in the low twenties because of the bumps and crosswind gusts.

When I turned around near the Transition area to start my second loop, I knew I was way behind my schedule. I stopped at an Aid Station to get more hydration and check my plan on the laminated card in my back pocket. It confirmed what I feared. The first loop took about forty-five minutes longer than expected. I had a lot of work left to do. I felt strong on the lower section of the route, but once I was back on the Beeline Highway section, the wind and incline again had a huge impact. I rode up with a little more focus, trying to make up some time.

The bottom of my left foot was starting to be a little painful. It wasn't cramping, though. It was as if the tissue on the ball of my left foot was getting crushed, and it was bruised. That was the part of my foot where the skin was ripped off in the previous IRONMAN event. The skin grew back, but the area was still tender. That was the point on my foot that was in contact with the pedal. I don't know if it was an issue due to my cycling form, but I focused on spinning my legs in a nice smooth circle rather than pushing down on the peddles. That part of my foot gets sore sometimes, even when I've been off my bike for a few weeks, so I suspect it's not an issue with my cycling form. Either way, it didn't matter. It hurt, but I still had a long way to go. There would be time tomorrow to accept the pain.

I was riding slowly, maybe 8 to 10 miles per hour, as I neared the turnaround point where the headwind and grade were the most difficult. When I made the U-turn to come back down the hill, I knew I had to pick up the pace. It was the same issue as the first time down; the rough road and road gaps were making my bike vibrate and hard to control. I did my best to come down with some speed while staying upright on my bike. I spent a lot of time coming down the hill, struggling to maintain control of the bike rather than being able to get as much speed as possible. As I rode down, I noticed the long line of riders to my left slowly climbing up the hill on the other side of the road. They looked like they were barely moving.

As I made the U-turn near the Transition area to start my last loop, I thought to myself, *This is turning into a real bitch of a ride, and there's still thirty-eight miles left to go.*

I stopped at an Aid Station after the U-turn to quickly grab some nutrition and give my left foot a break. I knew I would have to ride up as fast as I could and thought a short break would help over the long-term. I looked at my laminated card. I had once again lost time according to my plan on the second loop, but it wasn't as bad as the first loop.

I needed to make up some time. It was eight more miles to the area where I could pick up my Bike Special Needs bag. My plan was to stop there for a few minutes for a quick break and then ride the remaining ten miles to the turnaround at the top of the hill, take a quick break on top, and then come down as fast as I could. I wanted to break up the rest of the ride into manageable segments with a few stops to help me ride faster overall.

I went up as fast as I could. I was already out on the bike route for a long time and still had a long way to go. I knew I would be getting very close to the cutoff time late at night, and every minute I could save now would be important later.

I followed my improvised plan with several quick stops, which allowed me to ride faster overall. I went up the hill at a faster rate than my first two loops. I took a quick break at the top to relax my left foot and then got back on the bike for the last time down the hill.

The wind was blowing as hard as before, and my bike was vibrating as hard as ever, but I had to press it. I knew how long the marathon would take me, so if I didn't make up time on the rest of the ride, I was in danger of not finishing the IRONMAN triathlon before the cutoff. That was unacceptable. I had been down the hill twice already. I knew what to expect and just held on tight. Screw being cautious. It was the fastest I had ridden all day.

When I was near the halfway point down and coming off the Beeline Highway, I noticed riders starting their ride up on that segment. My bike ride was taking a long time, and they were at least an hour behind me. I didn't know if they would make it. I later learned that quite a few athletes either quit on the bike route or didn't make the bike cutoff time.

One hundred and twelve miles into the ride and seven hours and twenty-seven minutes later, I entered the Transition area, signaling the end of the bike segment. I didn't coast in. I came in pretty hot and rode as far as they would let me. The volunteer Bike Catchers greeted me, and one of them grabbed my bike as I dismounted. He was going to put it back on the rack where I picked it up that morning. He and my bike went left, and I went right. It was a fast handoff.

Throughout the entire ride, I got off my bike five times. The breaks were fast, just about five minutes each. I gave my feet a break so I could ride faster overall and broke the ride up into more manageable segments.

## TRANSITION TWO

After getting off my bike, I walked toward the T2 bags, which were all laid out on the ground in numerical order that morning. There were more bags left on the ground than I anticipated, meaning those athletes had not yet come through T2. Within thirty feet of getting off my bike, a volunteer had already delivered me my bag. I headed toward the men's changing area.

Earlier in the day, after the swim, I changed outside the tent. However, this time, I went inside and sat on a chair. There were about fifty chairs neatly lined in rows. Volunteers brought cups of water to all the athletes in the tent. After a long day on the bike, the service felt as good as at the Four Seasons. Although I was in a hurry, I still enjoyed talking with other athletes. The general consensus was that the bike segment was a bitch. While chatting, I kept moving. I dumped the contents of my bag on the ground.

Again, I brushed my teeth, changed my clothes, put on my shoes, and placed the remaining stuff back into the bag. I handed my T2 bag to a volunteer and was off to the marathon course.

From the time I dismounted my bike until I entered the marathon course, just over thirteen minutes had elapsed. It was my fastest transition, and I was moving quickly. There was just a lot of distance to cover, which added up the time.

## MARATHON

The route was almost nine miles long and required three loops. The first few miles were on a dirt and gravel path. They were welcome because they were a little softer than concrete but bad because I was breathing in all the dust that people kicked up. By the end of the day, my eyes were all red and irritated, likely from the dust and dry climate. There were a few short inclines throughout the course, with a moderate hill at about mile six. There were portions along the lakefront, in neighborhoods, and through parks.

The Aid Stations were about a mile apart and each of the farthest points on the route had one. Each station had its own theme and was staffed with very enthusiastic volunteers who were full of encouragement. It was exciting to pass by one because they were like parties with music, lights, food, and drinks. There were parts of the route through parks on relatively dark paths, and I could see the welcoming sight of a well-lit Aid Station off in the distance.

There were thousands of spectators along the route; many had music, signs, tents, and likely, a lot of beverages. It was particularly crowded near the Transition area, which was an entertainment area anyway, and the excitement of the IRONMAN event likely brought out even more people.

My legs and feet were sore. Due to the left foot injury from the previous IRONMAN triathlon, I had not been on my feet much over the past six weeks. About a third of the nine-mile route was on a concrete walkway, but there was also grass or gravel right next to the walkway. I walked on the grass or gravel as much as I could, making sure not to take any shortcuts because it was easier on my feet and legs than on the concrete.

There were a lot of athletes walking. Parts of the route included an out-and-back segment, so I could see the other athletes walking past me in the opposite direction. Since there were three loops and several out-and-back sections, there was a constant flow of athletes around the course late into the night. It felt crowded with athletes during my first two loops.

One of the great things about walking the marathon segment was walking and talking with other athletes. I met people on their first IRONMAN event and people on their tenth. I was also able to be in the moment. I was tired and sore but still able to appreciate everything going on around me and inside me. I felt very fortunate to have the opportunity to participate in the event.

I kept doing math and staying focused on my pace. Since the bike ride took so long and I had to walk the marathon, I would be cutting it close to the cutoff time. I brought all my own nutrition and only had water at the Aid Stations, despite there being a variety of food selections available. I stopped drinking anything at about mile eighteen because I was concerned that if I had to stop and use the porta-john, I would miss the cutoff time. It was only with about four miles remaining that I knew I would make the time cutoff at my current pace. Despite the two replaced hips, torn meniscus, and a sore foot, I would have run if I had to in order to make the cutoff time.

## THE FINISH

On the final loop, athletes were diverted onto a different route about a quarter mile from the finish. There was a long, straight road that led to the finish line. It was late at night, and I could see the bright lights and hear the announcer off in the distance.

It was an incredible experience to come down the long red carpet again. I slowed down and high-fived a lot of spectators. It was loud, and there was so much excitement, even close to midnight. It was an unforgettable moment.

No athlete passed me for over an hour, but for some reason, athletes behind me who were walking started running and were passing me as we got closer to the finish. The way I looked at it, I had just spent all day for this red-carpet moment, and I was going to take my time there. I spaced myself out from other athletes, waved, blew kisses, and crossed the finish line hearing my name and the call that I was an IRONMAN. Six hours and fifty-eight minutes after starting the marathon, I crossed the finish line.

A volunteer put a medal around my neck, and another handed me a hat and finisher shirt. I even remembered to get a picture in front of the IRONMAN triathlon backdrop, something I forgot to do at my first IRONMAN event. My total time was sixteen hours and twenty-seven minutes. I made the cutoff with thirteen minutes to spare.

## AFTER THE FINISH

After I finished, I stuck around for about ten minutes to watch other athletes come through. There's no better place to be than at the finish line of an endurance event near the cutoff time. You can see so many athletes overjoyed at their accomplishment, and the crowd gets even more electric.

Once I left the immediate finish line area, there wasn't much to do. It wasn't very crowded. There were no restaurants or bars in the immediate area, so it was pretty quiet. Athletes were picking up their bikes and bags and leaving.

I claimed my bike from the bike compound and took it to the triathlon bike transport area, which was right next to the bike compound. My bike was to be shipped back to the bike shop in the Houston area, where I had dropped it off.

I then picked up my T1, T2, and Morning bags and walked back to my hotel. It was the last time I needed to make that walk along the path between the hotel and the Transition area.

I didn't have anyone with me, so I had to carry everything myself. I don't recommend it, but it's what I had to do. My wife would have loved to come and support me, but she was at home with our kids. It was about 1:30 a.m. when I got back to my room.

## RECOVERY

I had a relaxing night back at the hotel. I showered, ate, and rinsed out my wetsuit so it would dry enough to pack in the morning. I then walked to the ice machine to partially fill a garbage bag that I had brought from home. I sat on the couch, turned the TV on, and put my feet into the garbage bag of ice. After about an hour of icing my feet and knees, I put on my compression boots to continue my leg recovery and watched TV for another hour. I went to sleep at about 4:00 a.m.

The next morning, I woke up at 8:00 a.m. I was a little achy, but it was manageable. Although my feet and legs were sore, I had no blisters. I guess it helped that I didn't sweat much that time around, so my socks and feet stayed dry. The climate was really dry, so it kept me dry as well.

After breakfast, I made some business calls and then packed everything up to get to the airport for an afternoon flight. Less than twenty-four hours after finishing my second IRONMAN triathlon in six weeks, I sat at my kitchen table back in the Houston area.

What started three years before as training was now over. Mission accomplished.

# 12

# GIVING BACK

At the time of my first hip surgery, I had no idea what to expect. I was hoping for the best outcome but preparing for the worst. I didn't have a frame of reference or a role model for what life could have been like with a replaced hip. I wanted more help. I wanted to have a conversation with someone like me who had already been down the same path. Every step I took along the way was in unknown territory.

As I recovered, I was able to engage in a relatively normal lifestyle and slowly returned to some of my previous activities. I routinely questioned myself, though. *Should I be doing this? Should I be participating in group bike rides? Should I be taking long walks? Should I be torquing my hips so hard when playing golf? Should my hips and legs feel like this?* I needed answers, but there weren't any. I had to experiment and learn on the fly. If something caused me pain or discomfort, I had to figure out how to modify the activity to do it pain-free or mitigate it as best as I could.

All the other people I met who had their hips replaced were older, and they weren't as active as I was before and wanted to be again. So, I had nowhere to turn. Everything in front of me was a mystery that I had to figure out.

I learned how to make my legs the same length. I learned why the hip on my longer leg hurt. I learned how to end the stabbing pains on the sides of my legs. I learned which stretches provided the quickest benefit. I also learned that perceived limitations were nonsense.

I wanted to share that information and all the information I learned going forward with people who needed it. I wanted to be the resource I needed when I was going through my hip replacements and recovery processes.

## JOINT REPLACEMENT ORIENTATION

A year after my second surgery, I was speaking in front of a group of patients at the Joint Replacement Orientation class at the same hospital where I had my surgeries. It was a monthly class for all incoming joint replacement patients. I sat in the class twice as a patient, once before each of my hip replacement surgeries. I volunteered to speak at the class after my initial recoveries.

I knew I had valuable information to share with the patients soon to undergo their own hip replacement surgeries. I usually presented last, after the nurses, case workers, and anesthesiologists. I spoke about my experiences with the surgeries, what I did in the days and weeks after the surgeries, and how I recovered thus far from each one.

The plan was for me to talk for about ten minutes, but it always ran longer due to all the questions from the soon-to-be patients. All the other speakers were required to be there. It was their job.

They often took a very business-like, even cold, approach with their presentations. I was there as a former two-time patient. I knew what the patients were experiencing because I was one of them.

The patients seemed to want more information from me than the other speakers. Because of my surgeries, I could provide a perspective that none of the other speakers could provide. What did the hip feel like? Was it difficult to walk? How long was I on crutches? What were the precautions to use before taking a shower? How numb was the incision area and for how long? When was I able to drive? What did I do for exercise? What problems was I experiencing?

I stayed until everyone's questions were answered, long after the scheduled time. Our conversations were usually carried out in the hallway after our time in the conference room was up.

I remember how apprehensive I was before my first surgery. I wish I had someone like me presenting at the orientations I attended as a patient or who I could contact with my questions. I knew no one who blazed the path I wanted. I wanted to be a resource for people about to undergo hip replacement surgery so they could understand the process better. I wanted to make it easier for them than it was for me.

The IRONMAN triathlon was not even a thought in my mind yet. That was still years away. I was only at a point in my recovery where I was able to help those patients facing what I had already faced.

I participated in the Joint Replacement Orientation every month for almost a year. The nurse, who was the Orientation Class Coordinator, had taken a different role, and someone new took over. They changed the format of the class and reduced or eliminated the speaker roles. The timing of the class also changed, and it no longer fit within my availability due to the demands of my corporate career.

My message back then was important to a lot of people. I know I helped hundreds of patients and their families, but there is a much larger group of people in need of this information. I would like to get back to helping joint replacement patients and answering their questions so they can have the best recovery possible. That is one of the purposes of this book - to be a resource for patients facing a hip replacement surgery.

## ENCOURAGEMENT

Occasionally, I meet someone who will soon be having one of their hips replaced. It's usually when I see a stranger limping badly and I ask them about it. That's a tough place to be. I was there. I offer them words of encouragement. Everyone needs a little pick-me-up sometimes. Depending upon how deep the conversation gets, I might share my story. I provide whatever value I can while answering their questions.

Few people over the past several years knew I had hip replacement surgeries. When I tell people, they are surprised, which I guess is good because it means my recovery with physical therapy was so thorough that I could move without showing signs such as a limp. I occasionally get requests from people who know me to speak with one of their family members or contacts who need a hip replacement. I know they are not thrilled about what they have to go through, but it's rewarding to me to be able to help them, even if it's just a little. What once seemed to be a tragedy or some unfortunate luck had become a gift, one that gave me the opportunity to help others by offering guidance they were unlikely to get anywhere else.

## THANK YOU PLAQUES

I am very grateful to many people for my recovery. I could not have done it alone. I waited years to come up with an idea for how to show my appreciation to the surgeon and physical therapists who worked with me and helped me through my recovery. After I finished the IRONMAN events, I knew exactly what to do. I had plaques made for each of them. On each plaque was a picture of me crossing the finish line, and the inscription explained that I had both my hips replaced and then was able to finish two IRONMAN triathlons thanks to them. My hope was that the token of appreciation would remind them of the wonderful work they do and the extent to which they impact lives like mine.

While my primary goal was to show appreciation, there was also a secondary benefit. The plaques are now displayed in the surgeon's and physical therapists' offices. New and potential surgery patients and those going through physical therapy can see the plaques. I hope the patients will gain some inspiration to work toward incredible recoveries, go on to live happy and active lives, and rethink any limitations they may have imposed on themselves. If I had seen something like that hanging on the wall when I was going through my surgeries and physical therapy, it certainly would have made a difference. It would have eased my concerns. Rather than exploring the frontier of my capabilities, I would have strived faster and more confidently for a higher standard. It gives me great satisfaction to know that patients coming after me, people I will never meet, will see the results that can occur.

## MOVING FORWARD

I've done a lot of athletic endurance events, and one thing they have in common are the amazing volunteers. These are people who choose to support the organization and the athletes. They provide things like nutrition, hydration and, maybe most importantly, encouragement. They have a clearly defined role of helping the athletes. Maybe the volunteers are participants in other events, but for one particular event, they volunteer to support others. It is such a pure form of giving back to others because without the support of the volunteers, the athletes would not be successful.

When I was younger, I only considered myself to be a participant. I never considered myself to be in a supporting role. That has changed over the course of my life. Now I know I have many different roles. There are times when I play a lead or a participant role. Other times, I play a supporting role.

When I push my limits or try something new, whether that's in an IRONMAN event or business venture, I take a participant role because I'm trying to accomplish something. When I was recovering from my surgeries, I was in a participant role. I've also been given the gift of being in a supportive role for others who want or need something I've already accomplished. When I have the opportunity to help someone, I aim to be the best support person or volunteer I can be. It's just as rewarding when I help someone accomplish something as when I accomplish something myself.

I understand that my supporting roles are more important than my lead roles. I want to be the best parent, husband, coach, student, teammate, family member, role model, or friend I can be. That is the way I give back.

## UNDERNEATH

Things are not always what they appear to be. It's easy to look at someone and fail to see what's underneath. That, to me, is the essence of an IRONMAN event. Athletes come from all walks of life and bring different skills and limitations. Not every athlete is fast. Not every athlete has the time to train. Not every athlete is free from injury. Not every athlete is good at all three disciplines—the swim, the bike, and the marathon. Not every athlete is confident. Not every athlete is ready. But each one of them shows up and faces the obstacles during each event. They put themselves on the line. They choose to be participants and not just spectators. This is life.

I loved finishing where I did at the IRONMAN triathlons. Although I didn't finish last, I was much closer to last than I was to first. That was fine with me. A finish within the allotted time is a finish. I followed my plans almost perfectly and worked within my available skills.

The great thing about finishing late at night was being around all the athletes as the time limit approached. I talked with some of the athletes and watched others as they grinded toward the finish line. Some overcame incredible obstacles to be there. By all accounts, some should not have even been able to make it to the starting line, but they showed up anyway.

These are my inspirations—people who have every reason not to be there but show up anyway and grind it out. They don't make excuses. They don't even let valid reasons stop them from trying to achieve a goal. They go despite the obstacles they face.

I root for people. I root harder for people trying to make themselves better, advancing their limits. For me, pushing my limits at the time meant finishing an IRONMAN triathlon, but for someone else, it may be finishing a 5K charity run, a ten-mile bike ride, public speaking, or saying "yes" to something or someone new. Whatever it is, we all have boundaries, and those boundaries can be expanded.

Over the past few years, I did things I didn't know I could do until I did them. Every story where I learned about an athlete coming back from an injury, a business victory following a massive failure, or a troubled personal upbringing that turned into a massively successful life provided me with the fuel I needed to come back from my surgeries and accomplish what I did. I'm not the first person to overcome adversity. I just added to the evidence for achieving possibilities.

# CONCLUSION

When I was lying in the hospital pre-op room, terrified of the first hip replacement surgery, I was there because I just wanted to be able to walk with my little girl. Completing an IRONMAN triathlon wasn't in my mind because, as far as I was concerned, it was impossible given my "limitation" or "condition". I was aiming low as far as my recovery and physical abilities were concerned.

This has been a long journey in the making. My hips were so bad I could barely walk ten feet, and every step caused severe pain, first in my left hip and then in my right. There were probably five straight years of hip pain.

After my initial recovery and completion of physical therapy appointments, I just kept going. I wanted to keep getting stronger and better. Once I was able to walk pain-free after months of physical therapy, a second surgery, and another round of physical therapy appointments, I wanted to know what else was available to me. How normal could my hips feel, and how normal of a life could I lead? Whatever obstacle I faced in the form of pain or mindset limitations, I overcame because I wanted more out of life.

Having a hip replacement (let alone two) wasn't going to negatively affect me for the rest of my life. I wasn't going to let that happen.

I could have been content with just recovering enough to go for walks. I see lots of people reach a certain level in life, whether in their careers, health, or relationships, and simply accept their station. They quit growing and let life happen to them. That's not me.

## KEEP GOING TO UNCOVER MORE POTENTIAL AND SUCCESS IN WHATEVER YOU DO.

When I had my knee ripped up playing hockey, I was devastated. I didn't really understand how bad the damage was or what I would be able to do going forward. I turned to something completely new, swimming, to fill the void. I was terrible at it. I was embarrassed. I did it anyway. I would not have joined the swim team and learned to swim the right way if it weren't for my knee injury. The benefit to me over my lifetime has been immeasurable.

## MAYBE THE END OF SOMETHING IS REALLY THE BEGINNING OF SOMETHING BETTER. THE WRONG THING IN YOUR LIFE MAY NEED TO BE CLEARED AWAY TO CREATE SPACE FOR THE RIGHT THING.

Before my hip surgeries, I would never have done an IRONMAN triathlon. It just wasn't something I had a desire to do in my earlier years. It was too difficult. I only started to have the desire to do an IRONMAN event after my surgeries to push the boundaries of my capabilities. Without the surgeries, I would have never explored how far I could push myself. I would not have done an IRONMAN triathlon. I would not have written this book. I would not have helped all the people who benefited from my story.

## WHAT MAY SEEM LIKE A CURSE OR UNFORTUNATE EXPERIENCE MAY BE A LIFE-CHANGING BENEFIT.

I can honestly say that not only did I have my hips replaced, but I also had my approach to life replaced. My automatic responses of "no" were replaced with "how would that be possible for me." My mission and approach to life have greatly expanded. I've learned that I'm capable of much more than I originally thought.

Based on my previous misconceptions, I had no business doing an IRONMAN triathlon. I wasn't the IRONMAN triathlon type. Soon after I signed up, I had doubts and fears. I felt like I was crashing their party. By the time my second IRONMAN event came around, I had all the confidence and resolve needed to be successful. I wasn't crashing any party where I didn't belong.

## THINGS IN LIFE ARE NOT AS UNATTAINABLE AS WE MAKE THEM OUT TO BE.

I've learned that you don't have to look like anybody. You don't have to act like anybody. You don't have to do it *their* way. You can just do it *your* way and succeed at an IRONMAN triathlon or anything else. Figure out a way to get it done. Do it *your* way. It doesn't make an accomplishment less significant. Put in the work and you can succeed—*your* way.

You can get knocked down and come back and still succeed. You can accomplish much more than you currently comprehend. Be open to it, and when you find something compelling enough, don't just make it a goal, make it your mission. I had all the excuses I needed to avoid doing an IRONMAN triathlon. I did it anyway.

## YOU'RE MORE CAPABLE THAN YOU THINK YOU ARE. YOU DON'T HAVE TO FOLLOW THE NORM OR BE A CERTAIN WAY TO SUCCEED.

I have changed over time. I used to want things like houses, cars, or vacations. Now, I want experiences, new activities, new people, and new achievements. I want experiences because they cannot be bought. You earn them by pushing yourself further than you thought possible. You take risks. You reach for something that you think is out of reach.

I recently participated in a one-hundred-mile bike ride. I rode 115 miles. Why? Because I had never ridden that far before, and everyone else was stopping after one hundred miles. That's what I'm looking for. I wasn't capable of that for most of my life, either in terms of fitness or mindset. Things change, though. I have evolved.

## WE CAN ALL EVOLVE INTO BETTER VERSIONS OF OURSELVES.

I want to know what's available to me and what it feels like to achieve it. I don't care if I don't have the skills or background right now. Maybe it's impossible today but it could be possible tomorrow.

## THE OBJECTIVE MAY SEEM BIG NOW,
## BUT YOU CAN GROW INTO IT.

Time after time, I experienced doubt and fear. I was scared of joining the swim team. I was scared before my first long bike ride. I was scared before my first surgery. I was scared before my first IRONMAN triathlon. Looking back, my life has been a series of training exercises for bigger and bigger challenges. None of those things concern me anymore. What's possible changes over time. I made it so. You can too.

Every once in a while, I think back to when I was lying on that gurney, being wheeled into my first surgery. I had resisted that surgery for so long. I waited and lived in pain because of my fear.

I don't wait anymore. Whenever I have pain or obstacles in my life now, I move past them. Doubt and fear have been replaced with resolve and courage. I'm on a mission to explore my potential and help you explore yours.

I didn't set out to accomplish anything remarkable. I simply wanted to go for walks with my little girl. I just kept going.

How would it be possible...

# TIME SPLITS FOR EACH IRONMAN TRIATHLON

| | IRONMAN Texas | Strategy / Plan | IRONMAN Arizona |
|---|---|---|---|
| Date | Saturday October 9, 2021 | | Sunday November 21, 2021 |
| Start Time of Day | 7:28:20 AM | | 7:06:05 AM |
| Swim | 1:30:14 | 1:30:00 | 1:25:28 |
| T1 | 0:20:08 | 0:20:00 | 0:23:14 |
| Bike | 6:40:07 | 6:40:00 | 7:27:16 |
| T2 | 0:22:49 | 0:20:00 | 0:13:35 |
| Marathon | 7:23:30 | 7:30:00 | 6:58:08 |
| Finish Time of Day | 11:45:06 PM | | 11:33:44 PM |
| **Total Time** | **16:16:47** | **16:20:00** | **16:27:40** |
| Time Limit | 17:00:00 | | 16:40:00 |
| Time to Spare | 0:43:13 | | 0:12:20 |

# BONUS #1

# TWELVE TIPS FOR OVERCOMING CHALLENGES

## 1. FOCUS ON THE NEXT STEP

When faced with challenges, we often look at the entire challenge and fail to see that it can be broken down into manageable steps. In doing so, the entire challenge looks insurmountable, and people do not even try. They are defeated before they even start. One way not to gain anything from an experience or a challenge is to not even try.

Focusing on one step at a time transforms a big issue into a series of small issues. Once we can handle small challenges, we can handle many of them as they come at us one by one. Work on the very next step and gain the skills and experience necessary to address that next small challenge.

Let's take this book, for example. If I looked at writing 60,000 words, it would seem daunting. I may never even get started because it's so overwhelming. By breaking it down into 5000-word segments and then even further into 500-word subsegments, the book, and the challenge of writing a book, become much more manageable.

Take the power away from things you consider challenges. Break them down into manageable steps and address them one step at a time.

You still have an ultimate goal, yes, but when you focus on smaller steps, you create many small, easily attainable goals. Guess what? The more you achieve small goals, the better and more efficient you become at achieving those goals and preparing yourself to address larger challenges. Those, in turn, become easier once you have accomplished a few of them.

Focus on the next step. It is distracting and dangerous to focus on the wrong thing. Imagine hiking up a mountain. That mountain is the proverbial challenge you face, whether it's your career, entire life, or some other shorter-term challenge. As you start to hike up the mountain, looking at the peak will leave you unsure of your ability to finish the entire climb, and doubt will start to creep into your mind. It will cause you to give up. It will defeat you.

Just like looking at the peak when you are only halfway up is dangerous to your success, so is looking behind you at the bottom of the mountain. You may begin to feel satisfied with how high you've already climbed or that you have reached a certain level of success. That may also cause you to quit. After all, why keep going if you have climbed up so high already? Don't get comfortable with your success by looking at how far you've already come. There's more to do.

Instead, understand the ultimate goal and make your plan to achieve the goal by taking small steps. Once you reach a step, keep going to the next step. Be persistent with small steps, and do not stop.

## 2. GET HELP—FIND SOMEONE SUCCESSFUL AND ASK THEM

Everyone faces challenges. You're not alone. Chances are, no matter what challenge you face, someone else has already overcome it. In fact, some people may be experts in your very issue. Still others may have indirect experience applicable to your situation.

Find help in the form of experts, coaches, or mentors. The most successful people I know or have heard speak all have something in common. They have mentors or a team of advisors assisting them in many areas of their lives.

I used to try and do everything myself because I thought independence was a sign of strength and getting help was a sign of weakness. I could not have been more wrong. It's a sign of strength to reach out for help. Someone who asks for help from coaches, mentors, or similar experts understands they have more to contribute, and getting assistance is the best way to overcome a challenge quickly and consistently so they can continue reaching extraordinary successes in other areas.

I now have or have had coaches and mentors in many areas, including legal, tax, real estate, martial arts, swimming, cycling, speaking, writing, success, and many other areas. Having someone guide me through difficult issues, including learning new skills, helps accelerate the learning curve and ensures I am doing the necessary things correctly to achieve success.

It is common for the leaders who can help you to have received or continue to receive guidance from others more experienced in certain areas. Let these people be your guides. You can move quicker and more effectively with the right guidance and help from successful people.

When you receive good guidance, follow it. Sometimes the guidance is not what you expect, and it may seem contrary to your current knowledge in an area.

I used to receive guidance to relax more and take time off. I thought it was contrary to my success because I was always taught to work hard and work long hours. As it turns out, when I take time off, I am more efficient when I return to address my challenges, whether they are work-related or physical. Taking time away gives the mind and body time to rest and refocus the energy needed to overcome challenges. I am very grateful for this advice.

## 3. SURROUND YOURSELF WITH SUCCESSFUL PEOPLE

We all have a team around us, whether we know it or not. More specifically, certain people on the team may be helping us or hurting us. The key is filling our teams, or inner circles, with the greatest people possible. Those influencers in our lives will either directly guide us with their advice, indirectly guide us by setting examples, or subconsciously motivate us to certain results, either good or bad.

Imagine having positive influencers and successful people in your life. When a challenge or difficult time arises, they may be able to provide invaluable advice to help you move through or around the challenge. Maybe you can even witness how they navigate obstacles, and just by observing, you learn and adjust your behavior when facing similar challenges. On a subconscious level, you may behave or make decisions in a certain way because that is how you understand your influencers to act and make decisions.

There are many benefits to surrounding ourselves with the most successful and positive people available. They will influence us to become better versions of ourselves.

Unfortunately, the same goes for the other side. If we surround ourselves with negative people or those not on the path to living up to their potential, we fall into their practices and life outlooks. The negative attitudes and lack of drive for success become our approach as well. It will take a great deal of energy and courage to break away from that group, but it's necessary to live the life of our dreams.

When I was training for my first IRONMAN triathlon, I didn't go hang out at the bars at night and hope for the best. I got up early and spent time with other triathletes. I wanted to pick up on their overcoming adversity mentality, positive attitudes, and rigorous training habits. Just by being around them, I became more like them. I wanted to fit in.

This same thing goes for other endeavors. If you want to improve your skills in an area or your ability to overcome challenges, surround yourself with people who have already done it and who are successful. A strong inner circle will keep you motivated, raise your game, and propel you to the life and goals you desire.

It's much more fun to be around people who want the same things you want. There is a sense of team and camaraderie. Position yourself correctly in a positive group and let them propel you forward.

## 4. HARNESS THE CHALLENGES YOU FACE

Lean into the challenge. Consider any difficulty an opportunity to rise to greatness, with past difficult times being the training ground for what lies ahead.

Learning to deal with adversity is such an incredible skill. It applies to any area of life. In fact, the adversity one faces may prove to be an asset or invaluable skill later on.

There is a characteristic known as "grit" that many people possess. It's the ability to continue toward a goal despite facing adversity. Arguably, it may be more important to success than talent, resources, connections, education, etc. That is why seemingly incapable individuals with no history of success can rise to greatness.

The key is to accept the challenge and go as quickly as possible into the resolution mindset. Ask yourself: *How am I going to get past this? What is necessary to overcome this challenge I am facing?*

We often like to take the path of least resistance, so we shy away from anything difficult. It's during the difficult times, however, when we grow. The difficult times are the fuel we need to reach higher levels.

I like to think about two circles, one small circle inside a larger circle, like a bullseye. The small circle is my comfort zone. It's where my activities and thoughts are on autopilot. The larger outside circle includes the challenges I face and my goals. The space in between the circles is where the difficulty lies. I refer to it as my Uncomfortable Zone.

I spend a lot of time in my Uncomfortable Zone as I stretch to accomplish new feats and learn new skills. The best part of the struggle, though, is that growth happens. Once the items on the larger circle are accomplished, the larger circle becomes the new inner circle, and a larger outside circle with new challenges and goals is added. The comfort zone grows to the size of the previous difficulty zone.

When I was going through my hip surgeries and recoveries, I faced challenge after challenge. By overcoming them, I was more prepared for other scenarios later in life. It allowed me to appreciate my capabilities, complete IRONMAN triathlons, and write a book about the process. Going through those difficult challenges has helped me to someday reach millions of people with my message of recovery and hopefully push their capabilities beyond what they once thought possible.

## 5. TAKE CARE OF YOUR BODY AND YOUR MIND

Life has a way of keeping people distracted. I prefer not to use the term "busy" because I consider it nonsensical. Having a lot to do is no excuse for not accomplishing what is necessary to reach one's goals. It's just a matter of being more efficient on some tasks and eliminating others.

If you could eliminate 10 percent of the tasks you perform and also become just 10 percent more efficient on your remaining tasks, do you think that could make a huge difference? I would think so.

Taking care of ourselves is the way to become more efficient. That includes taking care of our minds and our bodies.

Our bodies are the tool with which we accomplish tasks. A more capable body that can generate more energy, work more deeply, and avoid sickness can accomplish more. Such a body can even handle more stresses than an unprepared body.

Consider the following to gain a capable body. Eating healthy foods while avoiding unhealthy foods, getting an appropriate amount of sleep, and exercising regularly all just require basic decisions. Eating something healthy or unhealthy is a simple decision. We all know the basics of nutrition. We may not know the specifics about nutrition, but I suspect most of us know if meal A is more or less healthy than meal B.

If we are not getting enough exercise, we may be thinking about exercise incorrectly. It doesn't take spending two hours in the gym five days a week. It may be as simple as a five-minute workout at home, taking the stairs instead of the elevator, or parking a little farther away than normal and creating a few minutes more of walking at each opportunity. Doing these simple things consistently can have a huge impact on your health.

Think about keeping a prepared body with exercises that blend what you are already doing, and then add additional exercise when you have created more time.

The mind must also be strengthened and ready to accept challenges. Thinking positively and being focused on a goal are critical.

I participated in a difficult thirty-six-hour endurance event. One of the coaches for the event, a retired Navy SEAL, spoke to the participants before the start and shared his three rules regarding adversity or any problem. He said you have three options: (1) you can fix it, (2) you can mitigate it, or (3) you don't get to complain about it. Nowhere in those options was quitting.

Get the mind right and prepared by staying positive and focusing on the goal of a completed mission. This is sound advice for facing and overcoming any challenge.

## 6. CHALLENGES MAY BE PREPARATION FOR SOMETHING BIGGER

We were all young and inexperienced once. Our challenges were about equal to our ability to handle them. Over time, we faced bigger and bigger issues, but as we grew, our ability to comprehend and address those challenges grew as well. Our earlier challenges and lessons learned prepared us for future challenges.

The same goes for the future. What we face today prepares us for tomorrow.

Consider what it is about the challenge you're facing that is different from previous ones and what skills can be learned from it.

Maybe this is the opportunity you have been needing, but you don't realize it yet. Maybe a relationship has gone wrong. Maybe a job was suddenly not available anymore. These occurrences may be the paradigm shifts that put you on the path to realizing your full potential. A better relationship and a different role may be right around the corner for you, but if you hadn't been freed up from previous commitments, you might not have been willing to accept the new opportunities.

I once knew an executive from my corporate career who seemed to climb the corporate ladder with ease. As a matter of fact, he may have been promoted many times beyond his apparent skill set and capability. He often explained that for his good fortune, he only needed to be perfect between five and ten times per year, that people are too busy to pay attention to you all the time, and they only assess your capabilities a few times per year.

It was those few times per year—whether in a presentation, a meeting, a sales call, making a key decision, or in a moment of crisis—when you must be at your best. Those are the key moments in your career and your life. Let all the other obstacles fade away. Focus your energy on being at your best when it counts.

So, the obstacle you face may be one of the few times each year when you need to really perform. Experiences through the remainder of the year have just been practice for the significant moments of truth.

If you can address your next upcoming challenge, you can tackle bigger or similar challenges next time. You can never go back to not having the experience. And you can never go back to the previous limitations you placed on yourself. After tackling a challenge, smaller challenges (once seemingly big) are inconsequential.

It is true that once you climb a large mountain, overcoming hills becomes inconsequential.

## 7. BE LIKE WATER

Have you ever tried to contain running water? Water doesn't care what gets in its way. Water focuses on getting around obstacles. There is an incredible lesson in water. Like Bruce Lee and many others before him said, "Be like water."

Water is the strongest physical force. It is stronger than earth. It is stronger than wind. In fact, it is a well-known hurricane survival tip—you hide from the wind, but you run from the water. That is because water is much more powerful and damaging than the wind.

Water is fluid. It takes whatever shape it needs. It is not confined to this shape or that shape. It does what is needed to be done and transforms into whatever the situation requires.

Water is also relentless. It will continue to flow and erode even the hardest rock. It overcomes obstacles in its path. Consider the Grand Canyon. The rocks and cliffs did not grow up on either side of the river at the bottom of the canyon. Rather, the water started as a small stream on top of the rocks and, over millions of years, eroded the rock to gouge out a deep canyon. Water is relentless.

When facing a challenge, be like water. If you cannot go straight through the obstacles, look for ways to go around them. Search for the weaknesses where you can gain some ground.

If you are told that something cannot be done, look for all the ways it *can* be done. Someone else may give you a different assessment of the possibilities. There is always a way to move forward. Sometimes, moving forward requires lateral or backward moves first.

Be persistent. Have you ever witnessed how little kids ask for something? They don't just ask once. They are relentless. If they get a "no" with the first request, they'll continue asking for the same thing every few minutes. It's a beautiful tactic. That is exactly the kind of persistence we need as adults to reach our goals. Unfortunately, kids are often taught or punished out of this behavior.

What a disservice to the kids. Early in life, they may just want a toy, but later in life, they may want a raise at work or to close a sale. The same persistence they exhibited earlier in life, deemed a bad behavior, is exactly the behavior required later in life to reach one's goals.

## 8. PERSPECTIVE

Many times, our challenges are the result of a skewed perspective, which comes from being too close to the situation. We're in too deep and cannot see the bigger picture. It's the proverbial inability to see the forest because of all the trees in our way.

Years ago, I was working downtown in Houston. It was about thirty miles to where I lived, and I often commuted on the bus. One day, as I was waiting in line to catch the bus home at the end of the day, I was in a somewhat sour mood. I wasn't happy with my situation, my job, and the challenges at work. I was not having a good day. Then, I looked around and noticed people getting in other bus lines. A middle-aged man walked up to another line using a cane to guide him as he walked. He was blind.

My perspective completely changed. All my worries and challenges seemed insignificant compared to the challenges this blind bus patron faced.

I realized I had nothing to complain about, and the challenges I thought I had seemed to melt away. All I needed was a new perspective to start making positive changes in my life.

Consider whether you are facing a real challenge or if a new perspective would change things. Getting additional insights from others may be helpful. Taking a step back and thinking about the bigger picture may also be beneficial.

Before I was married, I used to get invited to a lot of weddings. I think it was because my friends, family, and associates were all about the age when people generally get married. Most of the weddings were large, extravagant events. Trust me when I tell you I had lots of fun at every one of them. Even though I had a great time, I kept hearing similar stories from the newlyweds after the weddings. They would say the wedding was over too quickly, it took a stressful year to plan, and they spent so much time with guests that they didn't have time to really enjoy the wedding as much as they'd hoped.

After hearing that story over and over, my fiancée and I had a new perspective and took a different approach to our wedding. Not only did we elope to Hawaii, but we had a sunrise wedding about fifty feet from the ocean. It took less than twenty hours to plan, and thanks to airline miles and hotel points, we were able to have our dream wedding and stay in incredible resorts for two weeks for less than $4,000. By the way, that amount included the entire wedding—dress, rings, flowers, fees, photographer, champagne, car, flights between islands, and food for the entire two weeks.

We believed that more time, money, and effort should be spent on the marriage rather than the wedding. Our perspective had changed based on the feedback we received from others.

## 9. APPRECIATE THE OPPORTUNITY

All the successful people I know and have read about or heard from have something in common. They keep learning new things. Many of them are successful in multiple areas where they had no experience.

How do they do that? They love the chance to create and do something new. They appreciate the opportunity they have by overcoming the challenge in front of them.

I have mentioned before that I have my circle of comfort where I operate and have a larger circle of stretch goals and new experiences. It's the space between the two circles where I grow so that the larger circle becomes my circle of comfort and where I create a larger stretch goal circle.

It's uncomfortable to be in growth mode because things are new and uncertain. Often, I don't know what I'm doing. I keep going through it, reaching for bigger goals, because there is a peace that comes with reaching for my fuller potential. I appreciate the opportunity to become more than I was yesterday and add to my skills. I love the feeling of growth. I gain comfort from being uncomfortable.

There has to be something about your challenge that you love. Maybe you could love the result, getting past the challenge, or maybe it's the people around you experiencing the challenge with you. Regardless of what it is, find something to keep you motivated to see the challenge through to completion.

When I was training for the IRONMAN triathlons, I had to get lots of training done in the pool. Do you think I liked getting up early, driving thirty minutes, and then feeling the cold water? Let me tell you: I didn't like that at all, but what I did love was being in the water. I love the feel of the water. I love the smell of the pool. I love seeing the sunrise as I'm doing my laps outside. The cold water early in the morning was uncomfortable but I loved being on the path I was on. I was doing the right thing and I knew it. All those little reasons I loved doing what I was doing made me capable and focused on overcoming the challenge and getting the swim training I needed to succeed at the IRONMAN events.

You can do this too. Find something to love and appreciate, and your struggles will become easier. You'll be able to grow your capabilities while experiencing even a small piece of something you love.

## 10. TAKE STOCK OF YOUR ASSETS

When I was hiking up the mountain at my first 29029 event, I was in some serious discomfort. I still had a long way to go to the top and then I had to take the gondola down and hike back up several more times. I was exhausted, partly because of the physical nature of the endurance event and partly because of the altitude.

My mind was not in a good place. I started making deals with myself and rationalizing why it would be acceptable to stop before the thirty-six-hour deadline.

I knew I had to pull myself together and put forth more effort, so no matter what the result, I could leave the event knowing I did all I could. I didn't want to regret not trying my best. What I thought to do to improve my mindset was to think about all the positive things going my way.

I took stock of my assets. The weather was good. My equipment was good. The support and camaraderie were good. The food was good. I continued to think about all the positive things in my corner, and I started to believe the mountain wasn't so tall and was manageable. I could continue. I found strength in all the good things helping me, and I continued until time ran out. I did my best at the time. But, most importantly, I didn't quit.

When I face challenges now, I consider what positive attributes or things I have going for me. What's helping me that I'm simply taking for granted? I start to stack up all the things helping me, and whatever challenge I face becomes more manageable.

When you find yourself in a challenging situation, consider everything that is working for you. Maybe you have the necessary experience. Maybe you have been through it before. Maybe you have a good support network. Maybe you are physically or mentally strong and can withstand the challenge.

No matter your challenge, you have assets available to you. It may just be a matter of experience or training yourself to notice them. They can be tangible, like specific tools or people, or intangible, like determination or desperation. Even the good and bad experiences in your past may equip you and be resources that help you overcome your current situation.

## 11. THE SECOND TIME IS EASIER

The second time around, making a tough decision or overcoming a challenge is easier. You know what to expect, so any energy you expended figuring things out or working in the unknown the first time can be spent directly on overcoming the challenge.

That is how it works with challenges. They are only challenging the first time through. Each time you face them, they get easier. Not only does the same challenge get easier, but getting past it prepares us for larger future challenges. If you face the same issue again, you already have the tools you need to succeed.

It has happened to me many times, including during the second hip replacement surgery, my second IRONMAN triathlon, my second 29029 event and while writing my second book.

Before my first surgery, I was terrified. I had so many questions because there were so many unknowns. I delayed the surgery as much as I could. Even after surgery, there were more questions. I didn't know if I was going to be mobile. With time, effort, and support, I overcame all the challenges. I was much more comfortable for the second surgery. Many unknowns had become knowns, so I directed my energy toward recovery and not my fear or concern about the future. All I had to do was follow the path I had already made for myself.

The same thing happened for my second IRONMAN triathlon. I was focused and well-trained for the first one. I double- and triple-checked my bags and my strategy. My bags were packed days before leaving home for the event. For my second IRONMAN triathlon, it was the opposite. The nerves were gone, and I was shocked at my level of relaxation. I wasn't concerned about the triathlon at all, but I was concerned about how unconcerned I was. I didn't even pack until the night before my flight to Arizona. I focused my energy on a good performance rather than worrying about everything else. I had been down this road before, and the second time was much easier.

There was also a striking difference between writing and publishing my first and second books. When writing my first book, *Renting From My 6-Year-Old,* I labored over many points in the writing process and then the administrative or back-end business side of publishing, including working with printers and sales channels, which seemed to move excruciatingly slow. I had to focus on every step. With this second book, however, the story seemed to unfold for me, and the back-end portion of the business moved almost flawlessly. Even if issues arose, I could easily address them and keep moving forward.

The second time around is easier. Whatever challenges you face are making you more prepared for future ones. Even if you are not successful the first time you face a challenge, you will still gain invaluable experience and be much better prepared to succeed later.

## 12. ORDER OFF THE MENU

When given options among A or B, create your own option and select C. Many of the challenges we face are because we only see (or are given) limited alternatives for resolutions. There are usually many more options available to us once we realize there is such a concept and we take the time to learn about the alternatives.

Have you ever gone to a restaurant and been given a menu? The menu is usually just a starting point for discussions. The establishment couldn't possibly put all their options on the menu, so they offer just a fraction of what's actually available.

When I was in high school and would hang out in a friend's neighborhood, a favorite place to get food was McDonald's. It was what was available and what we could afford. My order would always be off the menu, a double cheeseburger plain. Why, you ask? Because they would have to make it fresh. I would always see them cooking my new burgers on the grill, and I would get them piping hot. The taste and quality of the food were always better when I did that because they wouldn't be able to use an old burger cooked hours earlier.

There is always room for negotiation. The key is knowing there are options and taking steps to explore them.

When faced with a difficult situation, always consider that there are options not readily apparent. Seek the guidance of experienced individuals and prepare yourself ahead of time.

A lot of the options will be discovered through thinking about the possible actions you could take or through negotiation if other people are involved. Negotiation is a learned skill; there are many books, podcasts, and other educational material available to learn enhanced negotiation techniques.

One thing to consider is that negotiation is an everyday skill. Someone is not a negotiator only a few times per year. Negotiation, because it is a skill that involves listening, learning, empathy, and communication, is an everyday thing. Every communication we engage in is a negotiation. Maybe the result is better service, a discount on a purchase price, or more money in our pocket. The point is that negotiation, practiced daily, can lead to huge rewards when high stakes are on the line and we are facing a challenge.

# TWELVE TIPS TO SUCCESS FOR HIP REPLACEMENT PATIENTS

## 1. UNDERSTAND THE DIFFERENT TYPES OF HIP REPLACEMENT SURGERIES

There are different types of hip replacement surgeries, and each type comes with different risks and benefits. The entry point can either be in the front of the hip or on the side of the hip. The material can be different. There are components made of titanium, stainless steel, plastic, ceramic, or other materials. The length of the rod inserted into the femur can vary. These are all things to discuss with your surgeon.

When I first contemplated surgery, it appeared to be my last option, so I did extensive research on surgical methods. I saw three different surgeons before finally deciding to move forward. I was no longer deciding whether to have surgery. I was already past that. I was choosing which surgeon and, therefore, which technique and materials would be used.

Before deciding to move forward, research each of the surgeons you visit and have extensive conversations with them. Ask questions. You don't just want the surgery to get a new hip. You want the surgery to get your life back.

You don't have to hire the first doctor who says you may need a hip replacement. Get informed. Go with the surgeon and technique that fits your lifestyle and desired outcome. I hired the surgeon who answered all my questions and seemed the most interested in getting me back to full activity.

Another thing to consider is the degree to which the surgeon is in touch with the recovery process. How much physical therapy is advised following a hip replacement? Well, it all depends on the outcome you desire. If you just want to be relieved of the historical hip pain, then likely little physical therapy is needed. On the other hand, if you want to walk without a limp and regain full strength and mobility, then a more complete schedule of physical therapy is required. It would be beneficial to have that discussion with the surgeon to determine if you and he or she are aligned with regard to the desired outcome and extent of the physical therapy.

## 2. GO SLOW

I wanted recovery from my hip surgeries to go much faster. It doesn't, though. Recovering from hip replacement surgery is hard. It takes a lot of patience at first and then months and months of physical therapy. I say months and months of physical therapy because that is what I think it takes to get back to normal hip function. The initial recovery period should be taken slowly.

It's better to take your time and recover on schedule than to rush the process. Hip replacement surgery is major surgery. Patients essentially have a broken leg bone, the femur, that must heal. It's a big bone, so it needs time. It also needs time to conform to the inserted metal rod.

There is a lot of rest involved. I spent much of the first few weeks lying in bed, watching TV, or sitting in a recliner reading. I'm not very good at sitting still or watching TV for extended periods so these were torture for me. Give your body the time it needs. To get a little activity, get on your feet and use a walker to move around the house. That could be part of the initial physical therapy. You may also want to move around to keep your sanity.

Allow people to help you. If you have someone to support you, let them do it, especially when getting in and out of bed and up and down from sitting in chairs. Put your ego away and accept the help. Be careful during those risky movements because that is when accidents (falls) are more likely to occur. Do not try to do things around the house. It's time to be lazy. Chores can wait.

The last thing you want is a setback due to a fall or sudden twist. I have a good friend who had her hip replaced, and within a week of being home, she fell and injured the hip. She had to have another surgery to replace the hip again because the first one moved during her fall. I know it set her back a few weeks at least. Not only that, she had to endure the risks associated with surgery, including the risk of infection, sickness from being in the hospital, and any risks associated with general anesthesia.

Any movement you need to do, and you think you need to do it by yourself, is just not worth it. Let other people help you. There is a time to be brave and a time to be vulnerable. Recovering from hip replacement surgery, when mobility is severely minimized, is a time to be vulnerable and allow others to help.

## 3. REHAB

Not a day goes by that I do not do some form of exercise or stretching for my hips. I do that to maintain flexibility around the hip joint and ensure there is spacing in the hip components to keep the natural lubrication moving throughout the joint.

I described my Rule of Thirds in chapter 8, and it's so critical that I'll mention it again here. The consistent positive ability to use the hip pain-free over the long-term is a combination of three factors: (1) the surgeon's actions, (2) the initial physical therapy (including rest period), and (3) the ongoing maintenance of the hip and surrounding muscles through exercises and stretches. For me, that means stretching every day, keeping the muscles in my legs loose, and using a foam roller or a percussion massager on my quads and IT bands (i.e., the outside of the portion of the leg above my knee).

It's important to note that there is no end to the therapy. Exercise and stretching are daily activities. They may look different for everyone, but to promote flexible and pain-free movement, something needs to be done daily. The rehab should be incorporated into your daily life. I suggest about fifteen minutes of physical therapy daily.

The main thing to remember is that movement is critical. The bigger the movement, the better. For me, big movements like taking long strides when walking, walking upstairs two steps at a time, cycling, and big stretches provide the most benefit. I suspect that is because the joint is getting more lubrication with the big movements.

I have friends who recently had their hips replaced, and they neglect this critical part of the process. They rationalize not doing rehab because they say their doctors didn't prescribe any, or the only prescription for therapy was to walk daily. I think that is an incredible disservice to the patient and human body, both of which desperately want to recover and move without pain. The hip is a complex joint because not only can it move linearly as in walking, but it also can move laterally and rotate. The best rehab takes all these motions into consideration.

Walking is a good foundation to get the body moving and can be supplemented with simple rotational and strength exercises for a long life of pain-free hip mobility.

## 4. SHOES

Shoes are an area where I recommend getting the highest quality possible. Do whatever you can to get the best shoes that are comfortable and fit you well.

I recommend the best quality shoes possible because you will want a good cushion between your foot and the ground. In addition to the cushion, good shoes will allow your feet and toes to work properly as you begin to use your leg and foot muscles correctly again. Good shoes will also help with balance and traction to keep a firm footing when walking and moving around.

Most of the time, I wear athletic or golf shoes (even when not golfing) because of the cushion and comfort they provide. In addition, the shoes I wear are deep, meaning my foot sits down in the shoe. The deep shoe allows me to wear an additional insole in one of the shoes and still have a comfortable fit.

I wear an additional insole in my left shoe to balance out the length of my legs. Otherwise, I feel like I'm standing in a hole, and even a short amount of walking will make the hip on the longer leg side start to ache.

I recommend athletic shoes following surgery for at least three months for the cushion and control they provide. Hopefully, you will be able to do quite a bit of walking as you recover, so athletic shoes may be the best option. As you get further away from surgery, other shoes may also be acceptable.

When I suggest that athletic shoes may be your best option, I mean running shoes because of the cushion, control, and comfort. It's okay if you're not going to be doing any running. You can still wear these great shoes.

To get the best athletic or running shoe possible, visit a dedicated running store instead of a big box sporting goods store, department store, or online retailer. Again, it's okay if you're not a runner. They'll understand. You'll get the best quality shoes, great service, and meaningful advice from a dedicated running shoe store representative. Plus, you'll get to try on different pairs of great shoes and determine which fits you the best. Do you think these shoes will be way more expensive than one of the other retailers? Think again. These stores carry higher-end shoes than those available in other retail locations, so the quality of the shoes is higher, which means a better fit and more comfort for you and your joints. Plus, your surgeon or physical therapist may know which running stores have discounts for customers exactly like you.

After training for and finishing two IRONMAN triathlons, I've covered thousands of miles and gone through many pairs of running shoes, even though I was walking. I have even found the perfect casual and golf shoes. I've tried a lot of shoes, and I may be able to speed up your learning process. Connect with me at ChrisBystriansky.com regarding any shoe-related questions.

## 5. RECOVERING FROM YEARS OF MISUSE + SURGERY

Recovery takes time. You're not only recovering from the surgery, but you're recovering from years of misuse of the muscles in the legs and core. You may not have walked correctly in a long time, and getting back to that will take patience and work.

The surgery was intense. You were asleep, hopefully, but here's what happened. The surgeon, or the team, sliced you open near your hip, spread apart your muscles and other body tissues, cut the femur, inserted a metal rod into it, and inserted the cup and possibly a cup liner deep into your hip socket. That's a lot going on in such a small space.

Take the time to heal, and then get back on your feet and active again. There are different stages in the recovery process.

The first stage is healing. That means getting a lot of rest. It is the stage that takes time. Let your body start the healing process. There is no need to take risks, and there should be no pain due to movements. I'm not suggesting you stay in bed all day, but I am suggesting you move slowly. It means no reaching, no twisting, and no unnecessary chances of falling. The doctor or their staff likely provided some light exercises you can do while sitting or lying down. Do those exercises as recommended.

Get up and walk with assistance to be active. Take small careful steps. Getting up and moving is meant to reduce the risk of blood clots and scar tissue forming.

The next stage is the physical therapy stage. You may go to a physical therapist for an evaluation and to learn new exercises to strengthen the muscles throughout your core and lower body. Increasing flexibility is crucial at this point. Regaining flexibility is crucial so that your hips rotate appropriately as you walk or move throughout your day. Go to as many sessions as possible with a physical therapist trained in hip replacement recovery. That initial work is the foundation for long-term recovery and success.

The final stage is the ongoing maintenance of the hip. It could include strength exercises, stretching, rotation, and walking. The goal is to keep the hip fluid and the muscles and other tissues around the hip supple. Talk with your physical therapist regarding long-term exercises to get maximum comfort and life out of the hip. Don't rely on walking as the only form of ongoing therapy and maintenance. Walking will not take the hip through its full range of motion, and the muscles around the joint may eventually become stiff and uncomfortable, leading to pain.

## 6. BE BALANCED AND LEVEL TO REDUCE ACHES AND PAINS

While I believe the doctors do their best, they cannot replicate the exact specifications your body was designed for and that you grew up with. It's possible (likely probable) the new hip was not put back in the same exact position as a perfect natural hip would have grown inside you. To take it a step further, the length may differ from what your body is used to. Yes, I know sometimes people naturally have slightly longer legs on one side of their bodies, and if they grew up like that, the body has compensated and grown that way. But when a new hip is inserted and the length is different, the body cannot grow to compensate for the difference anymore. If you don't physically make an outward adjustment because the hip is in a new place, it may put stress on another part of the body.

For example, following the surgery, my left leg is now about four millimeters shorter than my right leg. I don't notice it much when I'm barefoot, but as soon as I put shoes on, I feel like my left foot is in a hole. It's that noticeable.

How did I figure out it was four millimeters? I discussed the issue with my physical therapist, and he measured me. He had seen the issue before. He had thin wooden planks that were each one millimeter thick. He simply added them under the shoe of my shorter leg until I felt like I was standing balanced with weight evenly distributed across my legs.

If I leave it unmitigated, the hip and knee on my longer leg start to hurt. If I wasn't aware of what was happening, I might mistake it for another physical injury or condition. I use an insert in my left shoe to compensate for the shorter length. As long as I use the insert, my legs feel the same length. I'm balanced, the weight is evenly distributed across my body, and I can walk without a limp and with no pain.

Another random pain surfaced on the outside of my upper legs. It occurred within about a year of my second hip surgery. The pain was so sharp that I thought I had broken my femur or the metal rod inside my femur had moved and was causing the pain. I even had X-rays taken, but they confirmed that there was no damage. It turns out that the problem was simply an incredibly tight IT band. The IT band, or iliotibial band, is a thick band of fibers located outside the leg that runs the length from the hip to the shinbone.

What I thought was an injury or pain related to my hip replacements was easily treated with stretching. That is one of the reasons I stretch and work on muscle movements each day. Ten minutes using a foam roller or a handheld percussion massager on my legs is all it takes to keep my IT band loose and pain-free.

If you're starting to feel pain in any area, it may be a simple matter of tight muscles or other tissues. By staying active, stretching, and maintaining your range of motion, you will take control of your health and minimize the aches and pains.

## 7. EXERCISE ALL SIDES OF THE BODY FOR A BALANCED RECOVERY

Remember when I said that recovery from hip replacement surgery includes recovery from the surgery and from years of misuse of the muscles and skeleton in the body? Well, the exercises and physical therapy following surgery are meant to get the muscles back to working correctly. You're not doing the exercises to help the bone heal. Yes, the exercises will help circulation and thus blood flow to the area, but they are primarily to help get the muscles back in line and firing with each other in a coordinated fashion.

Over time, before surgery, as the hip became painful and caused you to walk and move incorrectly, muscles and the skeleton on both sides of your body were affected. All sides: left, right, front, and back began to work incorrectly as the body sought ways to function in the least painful method. But moving in the least painful method may not have been the motion the body was designed to use.

Physical therapy, including exercises and stretching, was designed to get the muscles back to where they belong. If you're only exercising and applying the physical therapy to one side of the body, the side that had the surgery, then you're not addressing the negative impact that occurred on the other sides of the body from years of misuse. So, exercise all sides to promote a strong, effective, and lasting outcome.

Rotational exercises are also important for recovery and a return to a full range of motion. The hips can rotate inward toward the center of the body (medial rotation) and outward or away from the center of the body (lateral rotation). Ensuring that these types of hip movements are included in rehab exercises will promote a fuller range of motion for the hips and a return to a more natural movement.

That means building in the habits to give attention to all sides of the body. If you're strengthening the surgery side, spend the same amount of time on the non-surgical sides. Your physical therapist will hopefully stress that to you and make sure you work on all sides during any in-person therapy session.

It will be tempting to not only skip the physical therapy at home but also skip working on the non-surgery sides. I understand life throws a lot of distractions at you. I cannot stress enough the importance of taking a balanced approach and working all sides of your body equally. It will help your muscles return to proper functioning, allow you to walk without a limp, and promote a long-term, positive outcome.

One of the ways to make time to work on all sides of your body is to do the exercises and stretching while doing other activities. If possible, and if safe to do so, sit on the floor and stretch or exercise while watching TV, cross your legs while sitting in a chair, or contract (squeeze) your legs and butt muscles while driving. Your physical therapist should have recommendations for the perfect environment to perform exercises but should also have practical supplemental alternatives that fit into your lifestyle.

## 8. TAKE RESPONSIBILITY FOR YOUR RECOVERY

Take full responsibility. To get the best outcome possible, learn as much as you can. Shop around for your surgery, not for the best price but for the surgeon who seems the most excited to get you back to your desired activity level. Obtain second and third opinions from different surgeons. Research the different techniques, entry points, and materials before finally deciding upon the surgeon and, therefore, the technique and materials. Take control from the beginning by selecting a surgeon who fits your desired outcome.

Before and after surgery, do all the exercises the medical team provides. Attend any available orientation before surgery. Be patient in your recovery. Follow the advice of doctors and physical therapists as to when to start more strenuous therapy.

When considering different physical therapy options and a team to help get you back to your desired level of activity, ask the surgeon for recommendations while letting him or her know your goals. Be clear with the surgeon. Do not limit yourself to a simple therapy plan from the surgeon. Physical therapists are the specialists in this area of recovery. Use them to get the best possible outcome.

Research the potential physical therapists. Learn their specialties. You want physical therapists who work with hip replacement patients every day and specifically with patients who have had this same type of hip replacement surgery.

Do all the exercises they give you. As your strength and abilities continue to increase, do more exercises, being careful not to overdo it but enough to make significant advances. This is in the recovery and physical therapy stage, so it should be safe to accelerate the exercises based on your progress.

Take full responsibility for your outcome. Don't just let the surgeon do his or her thing, complete some minimal physical therapy, and be done with it, leaving the outcome to chance. Instead, stack the odds in your favor by selecting the surgeon with your characteristics and goals in mind and the physical therapists who will give you the attention and work necessary to help achieve your goals. Don't waste time and energy complaining about aches and pains along the way, blaming someone else for a less than stellar outcome. Own the whole process by taking responsibility for your desired result.

## 9. YOU CAN BE AS ACTIVE AS EVER

You can get to an activity level you have not felt in years. Rest, do the physical therapy, and set your sights on the stars.

When I visited with the surgeon who ultimately did my hip replacement, he initially told me I would return to a high level of activity. I didn't believe him. He gave me examples of people doing some amazing things. Still, I was a doubter. I wanted to believe him. I wanted to aim for the stars in my recovery, but truth be told, I just wanted to be able to play with my daughter and not be a burden to my wife. Initially, that would have been enough for me. However, my actual outcome and activity level surpassed anything I had heard or considered.

Believe it or not, you can be as active as ever. It took me a while to start to believe that. Toward the end of the therapy after my first surgery, I started to believe. The exercises were getting easier, and the discomfort was getting less and less. I was exercising more, even going back to the gym and doing leg exercises there. It reached the point where I was doing enough weight and reps that no one would have imagined I had hip replacement surgery.

I was walking a little, and it took about six months after my second hip replacement before I felt comfortable walking a few miles at a time. About a year after the second surgery, I walked while golfing for the first time in many years. It was about a seven-mile walk, stopping to swing and putting some serious rotational torque on my hips. I was a little sore, but it was a smashing success. A few days, mostly off my hips, and some stretching were all I needed to feel good again.

I was cycling within about five months of the first surgery. I wasn't concerned about the stress on my muscles or hip because cycling is a pretty smooth activity. I was more concerned about falling and the damage that could do. I simply kept my distance while around other riders. I was extra careful while unclipping my cycling shoes from the bike when stopping. As any cyclist will tell you, it's not too difficult to get your shoe stuck on the peddle and fall while trying to make a simple stop.

I was back in the pool swimming about six weeks after each surgery as soon as the incision site completely healed. I didn't want to risk infection. I used a buoy between my legs to avoid kicking but was able to swim without a problem.

## 10. BELIEVE YOU WILL HAVE GREAT RESULTS

Before the surgery, I was skeptical about returning to an active lifestyle. I believed I would have a limited lifestyle because of the surgery. I wanted to get back to full activity, but I was skeptical. I believed I would be less capable than I had been in the past. I put off my surgery as long as I did because I didn't want to face the limited capabilities I thought I would experience. After witnessing the recovery process, I realized I had the wrong approach.

Do not set a physical limitation in your own mind. Don't set yourself up for less than optimum results. You can slowly transform your thinking after getting through what I consider the toughest part of the surgery and rehab, which is usually during the first month.

Once you feel confident that your recovery is going well and you can return to a good level of activity, focus on getting all the way back. You can do extraordinary things like anyone without a hip replacement and live a normal life.

Your mind can start the process. Once you can walk without the assistance of a walker or crutches, start to think about bigger possibilities. Set a goal in your mind, and your physical body will accomplish it. Believe you can do great things and return to full activity.

Associate with active and positive people. Join local active groups and participate in groups of successful people. Surround yourself with people who want more out of life and aren't satisfied with sitting around waiting as they age. This will be a huge benefit because they will motivate you to keep going and adopt an active lifestyle. Those around you will be your support group, and they will push you. Even if you cannot immediately participate in many of the group's activities, having that connection with an active group will help keep you motivated to stay active.

The best approach is to have a positive mindset and set your sights on a giant recovery. Spend more time being active than being alone. Surround yourself with people who are successful and active. Locate a group near you of people recovering from similar surgeries. It's great to connect with someone who understands what you're going through.

Associate with successful people who have had great recoveries. Find groups. Connect with our group at ChrisBystriansky.com.

## 11. STAY ACTIVE

Take a 50/50 approach. Try to spend 50 percent of your time off your feet and 50 percent on your feet being active. Activities off your feet may include sitting at a desk working, watching TV or reading while on the couch, driving, or sitting in meetings. Activities on your feet, or being active, may include things like hiking, cycling, yoga, stretching, walking while golfing, swimming, gardening, working out in a gym, and many other activities.

Ironically, the actions that may give you the most discomfort are the small repetitive ones. Engaging in slight movements over an extended period may make you a little sore. The little movements may squeeze out any fluid between the hip components, resulting in a slight rubbing or grinding sensation. Think about standing over the sink washing dishes or loading the dishwasher. Those little repetitive movements may make you sore and cause you to notice the hip implant.

Even standing may be less disruptive than the small repetitive movements. The simple cure for those minor aches is to be active. A little stretching goes a long way. Remember, moving the hip joint to get some of the body's natural lubrication is very helpful.

It makes sense because the parts of the hip implant need to be kept lubricated by the body's natural fluids. Large movements that accompany an active lifestyle keep the hip implant in motion and flexible, bringing in more of the body's natural fluids. Small movements seem to dissipate or squeeze out the natural fluids, but the movements are not big enough to bring in fresh fluid.

The best way to recover is to have an active lifestyle. You can be doing things and keeping the hip moving without even knowing it. For example, taking the stairs is great. Once you're strong enough, you may even be able to go up the stairs two at a time, and it may feel wonderful because you're getting a little stretch with each step you take.

It's important to do some activities or a group of activities that include the full range of motion. Mix up the activities you do. Have fun. Try new things or activities you haven't been able to do in a long time. The idea is to move the hip joint in multiple directions, including (1) front and back (walking or stairs), (2) side to side (dancing), or (3) rotation out and in (golfing). Although these movements can be incorporated into your life routine, nothing beats the stretching sessions using the movements, hopefully, that your physical therapist provides.

## 12. STIGMA

It's really strange, but when I first had the hip replacement surgery, I was embarrassed. I believed, correctly or incorrectly, that there was a negative stigma surrounding people who had this condition and needed to have hips replaced. Maybe I felt the stigma because I was so young to have this type of surgery. I felt like I was broken or defective.

As much as I hated talking about the surgery when I felt people were just making conversation, I loved talking about it when people needed help. There were several occasions when I was asked to speak with someone's family member or friend who was having hip problems and wanted to get more information on the surgery. Being a resource and being able to help someone was very rewarding.

I could not have been more wrong with my whole stigma belief. I was simply dealing with the wrong kind of people to understand and appreciate what had happened. Over time, I connected with more and more people who had or were having the surgery. I felt part of a group of capable and incredible people. Even if I didn't know them, I knew there were people out there who had the surgery. They weren't broken. There was nothing wrong with them. It's just one of the things that happens to people, possibly because of previous life choices, diet, injury, genetics, or whatever.

I am not proud of my hip replacements, but I'm certainly not embarrassed anymore. There's no need to be embarrassed. You can accomplish a lot physically for any person, hip replacements or not.

People who go through this type of surgery are not broken. People who have faced any difficult challenge and come out somehow scarred or changed are not broken. We are all just people facing the challenges that life throws at us. If others don't see us that way, we just need to find the right kind of people who will support and accept us.

I suspect there are a lot of people with physical or emotional scars. I've concluded that we're all the same. We've all had to overcome or deal with some type of adversity. Getting knocked down by life is not what's important. What's important is how you get back up.

# EXTRA

This is my second book. I wanted to share my ups and downs with you to help you get back on your feet, literally or figuratively, and help you gain the confidence to overcome the obstacles in your life.

While writing this and my previous book, *Renting From My 6-Year-Old,* I had many other book topics and ways to help others come to mind. I believe in the pillars of health, wealth, and impact and I'm working on a few projects to help people achieve their goals in these areas.

I would love to hear from you. If you liked this book and want to stay connected to get the latest updates or release dates on new material, connect with me at ChrisBystriansky.com.

I believe many people want to make a better life and also create a legacy—to be remembered for something. I'm going to help them do that.

I've completed two IRONMAN triathlons and have terrific memories and a new definition of fitness. Now it's on to the next challenge.

I recently returned from a golfing trip to Pebble Beach with a great friend. He's in his eighties, and it was a bucket list item for him. I was honored to be there to see him accomplish it. It was also a reminder of all the practice remaining to get my game back in order. I'm keeping my fingers crossed for invitations to golf at Pine Valley, Augusta National, Cypress Point, or many other wonderful courses. There are not too many experiences that can match walking down a well-manicured fairway with a caddie. It's so peaceful. Plus, I love the smell of the grass. All my girls also expressed interest in golfing more, so I look forward to spending more time with them on the links.

If you have read this far, thank you for being a fan. I am truly grateful for you. I wish all the best in life to you.

Chris

# QUICK FAVOR

First of all, thank you for your time and effort in reading this book.

I'm wondering, did you enjoy it? Did it provide value to you? If so, may I ask you a quick favor?

I'm on a mission to help a million people reach their health and activity goals. So many people suffer and fail to reach their potential because they do not realize what is possible. We need to reach as many people as we can. Will you please take a moment to post your best possible review of this book on Amazon?

Reviews are a great way to help others find and purchase this book. Please also share the message of this book with your family and friends.

I sincerely appreciate you and any help you pay forward to others.

# GRATITUDE

Thank you to the following:

My wife, for being by my side and supporting me through all of this. I could not have accomplished it without your support. You gave me time and space to go do crazy things and train for them. Your love and patience are inspirational. I still don't know how you do it all.

My daughters, for your patience while I was away training. Hopefully, you'll find some inspiration in all this one day. Let's have some fun now. I'll take you for walks, bike rides, to the pool or golf course any day.

Dr. Stefan Kreuzer, for your dedication, expertise, training, confidence and steady surgical hands.

Dr. Sam Dalal and Rich Cearley, for creating an engaging physical therapy experience and helping me get the best recovery possible.

The entire staff at INOV8 Orthopedics, including Brandi Peace and Monica De La Cruz, for all the work you do to improve the lives of patients.

Corin Group for all your innovation and help completing this project.

The IRONMAN Group for organizing triathlons and offering the opportunity for people everywhere to become better versions of themselves.

Good Times Running Company in Katy, Texas, and their entire staff, for helping me get my shoes and gear right.

IRONMAN triathlon training partners Amanda Forner, Janelle Chitty, and Joe DiGiorgio, for the countless hours you made either fun or interesting.

Fon Deuterio, Michael Roberts, and all the members of Katy Triathlon Club, for all your friendship and motivation.

TriDot and the TriDot Podcast, for all the informative content and for supporting triathletes everywhere.

My team, including Terry Stafford, Sissi Haner, Kevin Tumlinson, Dino Marino and Honorée Corder for helping bring this book to completion.

Honorée Corder, again, for your ideas, guidance, and inspiration.

# ABOUT THE AUTHOR

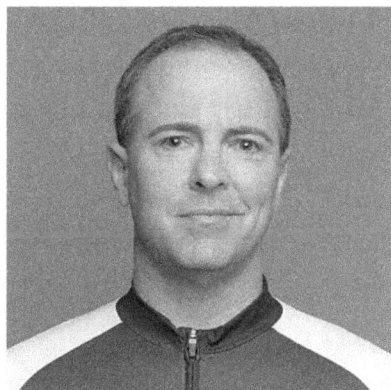

**CHRIS BYSTRIANSKY** (BY STRAN SKI) earned a world-class formal education after attending college, law school, and then business school. He worked in the corporate world for over fifteen years before finally breaking free to pursue higher interests, including investing in real estate, participating in endurance events and creating content to help people increase their health, wealth and impact.

He was very active in his teens, twenties, and thirties, participating in multiple sports, including baseball, hockey, volleyball, golf, swimming, cycling, and running. Chris underwent two hip replacement surgeries starting in his late thirties, the first in 2013 and the second in 2015. He then went on to complete two IRONMAN triathlons in 2021. He continues to be active today and participates in long-distance and other endurance events.

He is a husband, father, real estate entrepreneur, attorney, author, speaker, coach, golfer, second-degree black belt in Aikido, traveler, two-time IRONMAN triathlon finisher, 29029 finisher and more to come.

His first book, *Renting From My 6-Year-Old,* details Chris's transformation from an employee earning only a wage to an investor earning returns and the lessons he provided to his daughter to help her understand how to grow wealth and income streams. The book is a must-read for professionals not already generating extensive income from assets and parents looking to learn and teach their kids how to grow wealth.

You can find out more at ChrisBystriansky.com.

www.ingramcontent.com/pod-product-compliance
Lightning Source LLC
Chambersburg PA
CBHW032053020426
42335CB00011B/320